ENDORS

Dave's honest, practical and inspiring journey proves there is an optimism that is more than merely human. I am tempted to re-title it, FULLER FAITH (pun intended). It brought back warm memories of when he and Marilyn lovingly sat alongside me in a waiting room while my wife was in extensive surgery for a metastasized cancer. Their compassion for people is genuine and enduring. Romans 15:13 says, "May the God of hope fill you with all joy and peace as you trust in him, so that you may overflow with hope by the power of the Holy Spirit." Dave's life and words are an uplifting answer to that ancient prayer.

Mike Weber, friend and pastor

Dave's unique and vivid retelling from cancer diagnosis to "survivor" is both warm and inspiring! A gifted story teller, Dave walks the reader through the undulating emotional journey he faced—and we face—as cancer patients. Through it all Dave's story is a reminder that anything is possible—even in the most difficult of times and through the most difficult of circumstances—with faith and courage. Highly recommend.

Robert P Bickel, Sales And Technical Administration Manager

A Walk With God!

David C Fuller

"If you trust Me, I will carry you!"

My Journey through Cancer

A WALK WITH GOD My Journey Through Cancer

Copyright © 2021 by David C. Fuller
All rights reserved. No part of this book may be reproduced, stored in a retrieval system or transmitted in any way by any means—electronic, mechanical, photocopy, recording or otherwise—without the prior permission of the copyright holder, except for brief quotations as provided by USA copyright law.

Printed in the USA
ISBN 978-1-941173-49-7

Published by
Olive Press Publisher
www.olivepresspublisher.org
olivepressbooks@gmail.com

Front and back cover image: photographed by the author. All rights reserved.

Our prayer at Olive Press is that we may help make the Word of Adonai fully known, that it spread rapidly and be glorified everywhere. We hope our books help open people's eyes so they will turn from darkness to Light and from the power of the adversary to God and to trust in יֵשׁוּעַ Yeshua (Jesus). (From II Thess. 3:1; Col. 1:25; Acts 26:18,15 NRSV *New Revised Standard Version* and CJB, the Complete Jewish Bible.)

NOTE: The author has taken literary license to capitalize the word "Love" whenever he refers to his and his wife's Love for each other because his wife is a precious treasure to him.

All Scriptures are taken from the *New King James Version*. Copyright © 1982 by Thomas Nelson, Inc. All rights reserved.

Dedicated
to my precious wife, Marilyn

TABLE OF CONTENTS

Introduction

The Journey Begins

As an adventurous child growing up in a rural environment, I was always fascinated by the things around me. Seeking out and discovering the wonders ultimately led to the discovery that there are things that move which are crawly and slithery. These things provided a sick sort of enjoyment that only a boy could find fascinating.

At some point in time, I realized that these things are vulnerable and deserve more respect than just providing pleasure in vaporizing them with a magnifying glass. These things were created by God and contain the essentials of life. As I began to become more aware of this, I knew that there was a subtle yet significant difference in this thought process. If they were alive, then the opposite of that was death. This ultimately led to the awareness that there is finality in death.

In today's world, and to some degree in my era, there is this false sense that death is not real. Today, the games that kids play have a reset button which restores everything back to the beginning. Everything appears to be reversible, and in the past, to some degree, that was true in our imaginations. We would play war and pretend to be shot only to arise and fight another day. With the revelation that day that death is final, life took on a whole new meaning.

As we age and experience the loss of friends, family, and loved ones, this evolves into the understanding of our own mortality. Mortality finds its way into our consciousness and resides in our thoughts. What we do with this newfound knowledge affects our outlook on life, relationships with others, and ultimately our relationship with God. If we believe that our existence is solely based on the human form and that there is nothing after death, we look at life with finality. If, however, we believe that there is a continued existence after that last breath has been exhaled, we place a higher sense of worth on ourselves and others around us. This awareness is directly related to the ability to grasp this sense of mortality.

With this understanding about mortality, God, and my sense of vulnerability, I have found myself moving down a path which I always knew would come but never expected it to be so soon.

It all started when my wife, Marilyn, and I made a trip to Florida with some dear friends. After visiting my family, we headed south to a community called Venice. On this drive we came to the realization that we desired to be closer to my aging parents who, with my sister, lived in the Tampa area. Marilyn had already lost both of her parents, and we realized that if time was to be spent, it needed to be now. This understanding led to a whirlwind set of events involving buying a house, rearranging our careers, selling our existing home, and moving, all within a five-month period. Our lives were full of excitement and adventure as we had a sense of peace, looking toward our new lives. It was unlike anything we had experienced. All the components necessary fell into place. It was as if all the energies of the universe became focused on us and every challenge was resolved.

As a component of this move to our new life I, no we, decided that I should get a physical with our primary doctor in Indiana to establish a base line for the new set of doctors in Florida to work from. I have always been in excellent health and knew that this was going to be a routine visit with nothing to report. How surprised I was to hear from the doctor when he called to let me know that my Prostate Specific Antigen (PSA) levels were elevated to the point that he insisted that I follow up with a specialist. Two weeks before our move to Florida, my life was about to change. Still not sure if there was anything significant to be concerned about, I again drifted back to that moment in time where I became aware of my own mortality. Not that I was fretting over the outcome or even obsessed with it, but rather just aware.

God is amazing. But as we are going through life with its seeming randomness, we typically wonder what He is thinking or even if He is there. In hindsight, we can see that His presence is always visible. In my case, it is crystal clear to me. Several years prior to this decision to realign our lives, we became uncomfortable with our church relationship. This led us to search for a new beginning to continue our spiritual growth process. Ultimately, we landed with a small group of believers who were seeking to find true and honest worship. We found our spiritual home and welcomed it with open arms. They also welcomed us, and it was as if we had always been connected. One of the areas of focus we embarked on was centered on the ministry of Jim Richards out of Huntsville, Alabama. Jim's ministry was and is inspired in connecting with the nature of God and all the blessings and truths He grants us. One of these areas of focus lies in the understanding that there is a life force from God inside all of us, and that we have the ability to embrace this loving force for our own source of energy. In it we can, through God's blessings, face the challenges of life with a confidence and understanding of their outcome without fear or anxiety.

As I was presented with the news of the elevated PSA levels, I knew that this was going to be a journey which I had never experienced before. Because of the path God had me on to this point, I had a peace about the situation and knew what the outcome would ultimately be, but did not know how the journey would unfold. I knew that whatever the journey was going to be, that Marilyn and I would walk it together with God by our side, and that with the knowledge of our relationship, we would see it through. The understandings that Jim's ministry had imparted to us were and are invaluable. How were we to know that when we went looking for a new church family, God was preparing us for a future challenge? With this understanding, I will attempt to record the events of our journey. We know the destination and know the road may be bumpy, but with God by our side, we will walk it with confidence.

PHASE I

DISCOVERY

INFORMATION

ACTION

Chapter 1

Open the Gates

August 13, 2014

After visiting the doctor for a routine physical two days prior to and in anticipation of getting everything together for our transition to our new lives living in Florida, I was doing what I always do on a Thursday morning. I was busy tying up loose ends at work, repairing a roof, packing at home, and making arrangements for the upcoming sale. Then I received the call from the doctor. It wasn't an earth-shattering call but more of a matter of fact conversation.

"The results of your PSA (Prostate Specific Antigen) screening came back, and they were elevated. The reading of 26 is alarming and you need to schedule an appointment with a specialist for further review."

Those simple words were followed up with a conversation about whether I should wait until after the move and new doctors are established or do I need to begin the process right away in Indiana before our move. In the end, we, no I, decided that it would be wiser to begin the process complete with the new set of doctors who would ultimately be responsible for the care and potential treatments.

Sometimes it takes a while for information to be absorbed. This was one of those times. I went on about my business at work, mulling over the conversation. Although it was never spoken, the word "cancer" is almost always in the conversation when discussing the prostate. For some reason these two words have become conjoined in a way that it is unusual not to hear them spoken together. After clearing the items on my immediate agenda, I called Marilyn to let her know. We are both very positive people and have the ability to work through issues together; still I could sense concern in the conversation.

After getting home that day, we both began the process of exploring the meaning of the results. There are various websites online that talk about the medical evaluations and prognosis of elevated PSA levels. None of these paint a flowery picture, and inevitably they all place a high probability of cancer into the equation. Although they were not reassuring, they were very informative. During the early searches, I was focused on understanding what the results meant. These searches went something like this: "Elevated PSA Levels"; "Understanding Elevated PSA Levels"; "Prostate Cancer"; "Prostate Cancer Treatments"; *"Prostate Cancer Survivors."*

I put the last one in italics because it was not part of the search process. I never at this point firmly connected my condition with prostate cancer and, therefore, never identified with the word "survivor." Looking back, I find that this was done not out of denial but rather out of a positive attitude, which I have always possessed. I'm not saying that this is the correct way of looking at challenges in our lives, but rather my way. I have been blessed with the ability to not jump to conclusions in my life, but rather to wait until the facts are presented and then formulate a plan through the situation. Some people call this naive, but I choose to call it informed.

Marilyn's take on this is that it comes across as emotionless. We continually have conversations about how I don't show emotions, and she is mostly correct. The reality is I don't show emotions outwardly, but that doesn't mean I don't feel them. I'm not sure which path is better, to show or not to show. I only know that the process I go through works for me and that for those who process differently, I should communicate better.

Next came the waiting game, going about life by doing what is required. Our lives were very busy at that time, as the move date was quickly approaching. Days would begin at 5:30 in the morning and our heads would hit the pillow around 10:30 at night. It was during one of those short rests that I began having a simple dream. Picture a vision of either the morning dew evaporating into a mist or when an afternoon shower hits a hot sidewalk and gentle mist rises as it evaporates into thin air. This dream of that vision happened over repeated nights. As a believer that our dreams are connected to unresolved conscious issues, I soon realized that this was a representation of the challenge I was facing. Whatever was causing the elevated PSA levels in my body was not here to stay. It will simply slip away with the mist. Once this revelation became apparent, the dream went away like the mist only to be replaced with a new vision.

As most who know me understand, I am an individual who embraces the cards I have been dealt. I believe they have been given to me for a reason and that the dealer, God, put them here on purpose to help me to grow, to humble me, to provide me wisdom, or simply for His amusement. Most likely not the latter. Whatever the case, we are destined to face them head on with Him by our side, sometimes guiding, sometimes consoling, and sometimes laughing.

I share this analogy, knowing that we all have a favorite artist whose paintings or sculptures inspire us. Now imagine that if you were a proud owner of, let's say, a Monet, and you would step back, grab a paint brush, and declare, "I think it needs another brush stroke here," as you swiped across the painting. It would immediately lose its value, as you would have transformed it into something the artist did not intend. I look at the human body in the same way. God is the artist and for all the twists and turns we take, we are living out His masterpiece. No additional brush strokes are required.

A new dream emerged out of the mist; pardon the pun. In this dream, I was enjoying life with my friends and loved ones when I realized that I had a tattoo. It was located on my right shoulder and it simply said the word "**SURVIVOR.**" The next morning, I woke up and as we were getting around, I shared with Marilyn, "I am getting a Tattoo." She looked at me with amazement. The normal me didn't ever have any desire to adorn myself with a tattoo. In fact, I was the person who talked others out of getting tattoos, so for these words to come out of my mouth, Marilyn was caught off guard. When I explained the context of the dream and its meaning, she reluctantly embraced the idea.

As that concept crept into our minds, we realized the significance of the statement, that "in order to be a survivor, you must survive from something and this something must be real." This something will have to be profound enough that it would inspire you to reset your value system and allow for a tattoo. However, as we followed the dreams, we surmised that this "something," while serious enough that it needed to be addressed, will eventually evaporate like the mist and, in the end, I will be a survivor. The journey ahead will, in fact, be rough. There will be bumps and turns along with potentially lost maps, but the journey will be completed. This is the great news, "I WILL GET A TATTOO."

I was raised in a small burg in southwest Michigan. It was situated on the border of Indiana and, because of its remoteness, we had an Indiana address. Back then the focus was not so much on the who's but more on the how's. It didn't matter that the mail carriers had to cross the state line to deliver mail. It only mattered that there were people who needed mail service and they were capable of fulfilling that need. This simple concept became the basis of a belief system that I carry today. We all have needs that should be fulfilled, and if we are able to play a part in that, then we should. Instilled in my family was a quiet conservative presence along with an acceptance of who we are and who we can become: Nothing precocious but proud. Strong disciplinarian parents who we knew loved us. An understanding that there is a God who loves us no matter our circumstance and who is waiting with open arms.

Marilyn also grew up in a small town but located in northern Indiana. Her life was similar yet vastly different from mine. Her family was Old Order German Baptist, who wore traditional clothing similar to the Amish. Dresses, no radio or TV, and Sunday church were all part of her childhood routine. This lent itself to a strong conservative belief system and an even stronger love of family. While her family was solid and connected, mine was independent and distant. In either case, we had a very similar belief system instilled in us which became our set of values.

This may have contributed to the attraction that drew us together. We met through a mutual friend and coworker who unwittingly brought us together. We had each been in a previous marriage, which we entered into believing it would be long term. Ultimately, that desired reality did not play out. For me, there came a realization that I was simply biding my time, growing more distant until the inevitable moment when I knew it would end. Marilyn's story was different. Her relationship became abusive and, like me, she also didn't want to give up on the promise she'd made in her vows. However, there comes a time when the pain of the situation becomes too great to bear.

Both of us were in need of something stable, comforting, and loving in our lives. What started off as an acquaintance moved into a solid friendship. From there we began to confide in each other, sharing our pain and disappointment along with our desire to find someone we could share life with. As this friendship blossomed, we realized that the answer was simply standing in front of us. The friendship quickly blossomed into a deep love and respect and, ultimately, our marriage. The key to our relationship is in our friendship and respect that came first. We both realized that this was missing in our previous marriages. Now, I can say marrying Marilyn was the wisest decision I made in my life. As this journey before us began to unfold, I desperately needed someone who would walk by my side through the valleys and mountain tops. I am truly blessed and honored to be able to call her my wife and friend.

As mentioned before, the next few weeks were filled with preparation activities. There was so much to do that there was little time to think about the different scenarios. We simply had to trust in God and continue to do what we needed to do for the move. In reality, this was probably the best thing for me. When I would take a moment to run the possibilities through my mind, I would begin to sink into a light depression. It is easy to play out the worst case scenarios in your mind, and, knowing that where you are focused is the direction you will take, I could not afford to let the bad paths become my area of focus.

The immediate area of focus for us was the move we had begun. We had managed to sell the vast majority of our accumulated possessions. Our transition to the Florida home involved a significant amount of downsizing. Forty-three hundred square foot home, twelve and a half acres of land, a pole barn, and all the stuff to support it would not fit into a retirement villa. So, during this time of the unknown, we were preparing for two journeys. One as a physical move, which we have done before, and another into an unknown landscape—the world of the medical field. With everything sold except the chosen treasures we would take, we loaded the truck and headed south. Arriving safely, we were able to settle into our new home quickly, as it came fully furnished and stocked. Little did we know that this would be a blessing in disguise.

During the pre-trip preparation time, I heeded the advice of my family doctor and consulted with my sister to determine which doctors in Florida would be best suited for my condition. She had assumed the role of Care Giver Advocate for our aging parents and had extensive contacts with a host of providers. Her no-nonsense method of discerning the facts and keeping everyone focused had proven to be a valuable asset. Her background as a librarian lends itself well to doing research and disseminating information. On her advice, we contacted a local urologist who set up my appointment for one week after we arrived. This would give us time to at least become partially settled before we began phase I of the journey. I am calling this the *discovery phase*.

While we were waiting for the appointments to begin, and in the little bit of free time we had, we did some research. This provided us with a general knowledge of the condition, possible causes, possible outcomes and processes for the different scenarios. When the time came, we went to the doctor's office to start the process. We met the doctor and gave him the previous lab results. After reviewing them, he acknowledged that my PSA level of 26 was extremely concerning and that we should immediately start a complete evaluation. These simple words had a profound impact. One required test was a Digital Rectal Exam (DRE). This is where the doctor dons a glove, lubricates it well and proceeds to shove a finger up your ****. This procedure allows him to feel the prostate and determine if there is any deformity or hardening. Unfortunately, during this exam, he did feel both. There was a slight deformation of the prostate and some solidification. Both of these can be expected in a male as a normal process of aging; however, they can also be indicators of more serious conditions.

Next came the blood test for a follow up PSA screening. This is a normal step in the evaluation process. Being the ever present optimists, we also had requested it as confirmation of the elevated PSA level to eliminate the possibility of a false positive reading on the first test. After discussing the results of the exam, it was decided that a prostate biopsy would be the next step. This further defines the condition and is necessary in determining the next steps. An appointment was set for one week from the initial visit, and we were sent on our way to the lab for blood to be drawn. Getting blood drawn is a routine procedure for me. Ever since I can remember, I have never had an issue with needles. Growing up in a rural environment, along with an adventurous spirit, lent itself to significant opportunities for needles to be poked into me, but that is another story.

The interesting thing about this appointment is more in the lab itself than in the process. We had never been exposed to the independent lab style of business before. It was a small strip-mall style of a professional building, sitting behind a set of stores and gas stations off a side road. Where we entered and signed in, there was a reception area, a receptionist, and a few other people waiting for their appointments. After registering, I was called back to a crowded waiting room. This was more of a production line environment than the medical environment I was used to. I guess this is the new norm when you live in a geriatric state like Florida.

With blood drawn, again we move into the waiting stage. Somehow, this is the most painful part. If you let it, this is when your mind begins to play out the scenarios of *what ifs*. For me, the hardest thing was resisting the desire to begin more research, as I am a "get the facts" guy. When a subject comes on my radar, I will begin the process of understanding all that I can about it, so I will be prepared for any future decision. This has served me well in the past when it comes to making purchases, fixing things, and just obtaining general knowledge. But with health issues, you almost need to protect yourself. I don't mean that you should bury your head in the sand, but the information available is typically negative. Even the searches you do online talk about risks, treatments, outcomes, and side effects. These are all focused on the negative aspects of a condition.

A very important precept I have learned over the years is that you will go where your mind is focused. If the information I'm feeding on is all negative, then I will naturally gravitate toward being scared and depressed. Without sufficient positive counteractive information available, the best way for me to handle this is to absorb only a little of the negative and allow my attitude and value system sufficient time to add the positive. This is not denial but rather a defense mechanism. So, the process for me is to do a little research and then sit back. This process has helped me stay focused on the victory and not get caught up on the journey. During this time, it was apparent to me that I must protect my attitude and allow the earlier vision God had given me to become my reality.

Having decided that the conditions warranted the need for a biopsy, the next appointment was scheduled. As the date grew closer, I became more anxious. This was for two reasons. The first was the procedure itself. Knowing that the doctor was going to remove tissue from my body didn't bring a comforting feeling. Having read a little about it, I knew that it would be okay, but the thought of him coring an organ was disconcerting. The second was the anticipation of the results from the PSA re-screening. Hoping the first screening was a false positive, it was my desire to be informed that the PSA levels were normal, and the first lab had made a mistake. Unfortunately, the results from the lab indicated that the level had increased to 32. This could be within the margin of error or the differences in the testing facilities but, none the less, they were consistent. This meant that the condition was real albeit the cause not firmly identified.

The attending nurse and doctor were great. I have found that my source of apprehension typically comes from not knowing. This has been true for me all my life and most likely true for you. Reading about a prostate biopsy is one thing, but experiencing one is a totally different story. As the procedure began, they talked me through the entire process. From the preparation, through the procedure and the expectations during the recovery, all was meticulously communicated. Knowing what was happening helped keep a sense of peace and control because, from my vantage point, it was hard to see anything. However, I admit there were times when I felt that, for what they were describing, maybe ignorance would have been better. None the less, we slid through the process as expected. Setting up the appointment for the next visit to officially chart a course of action felt good, as I now had a time frame of when answers would come. Even though we didn't know what those answers would be, simply having a time frame provided comfort. The challenge was again in the waiting. The lab needed seven to ten days to process the samples and return the results, so the next appointment was set for ten days. Home from the procedure, things were fine as the local pain killers were doing their job.

Given instructions that the recommended pain management should be Tylenol, we ensured there was indeed some in the house as we settled in. As the anesthesia began to wear off, I realized why they used a local, not that I had any doubts anyway. The pain levels escalated to a point where I took two pills and relaxed, trying to get comfortable. The rest of the day was uncomfortable but tolerable.

Additional instructions to drink lots of water were also given. The biopsy process pierces through the prostate and into the urethra. This causes minor bleeding which can clot and block the flow of urine. To remedy this, there is no substitute to simply flushing it all out. So, every hour I drank 20 ounces of water, which definitely kept me from being a couch potato. Up every 10 minutes to go relieve myself reminded me that this was a surgical procedure. Even as I went to bed, there was a discomfort which miraculously improved during the night. Waking up the next morning with only a little soreness was a welcome feeling, and as the day progressed, the discomfort fully disappeared.

During this process, we have been careful not to involve a lot of people. The facts were indicating a potential positive outcome, but still there was a doubt. After the biopsy, we felt it was appropriate to bring some close people into the loop. I have never been a "poor me" kind of guy, so we began to choose who we would inform and when. Three people who were informed from the beginning were my sister and my two sons. Jeff is technically my employer, but we have developed a strong relationship over the years. I value his friendship, concern, and insight greatly. Meeting Jeff for the first time when he was twelve years old and working part time for the company he now owns, we quickly took on the roles of dad and son, at first jokingly but during the latter years more traditionally. Now granted, I never paid child support to his mother as we joked about, but I loved him like a son, so technically he became one.

Josh, on the other hand, is my son. He is a wonderful young man who has a sensitive side. Ever since he and his mother became a part of my life, I have been blessed. My relationship with him is and will always be strong, as we both, at least I, desire and enjoy it tremendously. Josh does have a tendency to worry about things though, so to inform him about a potential problem would likely place undue stress in his life. Still, he is a significant part of my life and we felt it would be unfair for him not to know. Sharing the facts as we knew them and cautioning him not to jump to conclusions, we began the journey together.

The waiting can be agonizing. We must remain vigilant when it comes to our thoughts, as we can drift effortlessly into the "WHAT" game. What caused this? What are we going to do? What are the results? WHAT, WHAT, WHAT....? This mind game serves as a useful tool when it comes to evaluating options, but it can become destructive when you allow it to infiltrate and consume the majority of your thoughts. Questioning and seeking wisdom is a good thing, but it can lead to doubts.

Chapter 2

Ownership and Choices

Whenever I have been faced with a challenge, whether it is building, fixing, creating, or accomplishing something, I will look for the tools around me to help in the process. When faced with the challenge of prostate cancer, I again found myself searching for tools. To date, the external tools I have identified that can be directed at the problem are the medical profession with their knowledge, wisdom, experience, skills, drugs, and treatments.

The internal tools that I can bring to the table are attitude, wisdom, ownership, commitment, and faith. It is important for me to stay focused on the "what can I do" part of the equation and to remain an active participant in the external tools but not get caught up in them. This being said, the tools that I have, which will affect the outcome more than anything else, exist in my belief system. What I believe, and the faith I apply toward it, will determine the journey and outcome.

I will take ownership of the fact that I have prostate cancer. There will be no denying the evidence. This is very important in the process. If I simply go about life with my head in the sand and ignore the condition, then I am in fact resolving myself to the external forces and their will. This would be a very convenient way of approaching the problem, as I could easily begin the blame game. Everyone and everything around me are to blame and, therefore, I can justify feeling sorry for myself. This leads to a very bitter point of view and, most importantly, leaves no room for God to work. If I continue to deny the existence of the cancer, then God cannot heal and comfort from something that doesn't exist. Only through the acceptance of the condition can I unleash God's involvement towards its solution.

I will continue to stay informed and educated. I have learned that God will use the tools in his tool chest toward a solution. Bruce Wilkinson, in his book *The Dream Giver*, makes reference that God is always preparing us for future problems. I cannot be so selfish as to think that God is only preparing me—but rather He is preparing all. As we continue to seek greater understandings of our existence, the information we have available evolves. It is imperative that I continue to seek those around who are being prepared to solve a problem like prostate cancer. The advancements and understandings in the medical profession continue to amaze me. Almost every day there is a new discovery about a condition, which places a glimmer of hope in the lives of the stricken. There are cures and advances being made in the field of oncology that are being learned and released every day, and it is my responsibility to assist the medical field in bringing awareness to my team.

I will continue to keep my attitude in check. So many times I have been close to individuals whose attitudes are defeatist. Again, I believe this stems from the inability of these people to attach ownership to the problem. If they are merely spectators in life, then everything is beyond their control. If they can control nothing, then there is no use to try, and life becomes hopeless. If life is hopeless, then they might as well succumb to the inevitable and simply wait for the outcome to materialize.

This attitude of helplessness is totally foreign to me. My attitude toward life lies in an understanding that ALL things are gifts from God. This attitude of appreciation lends itself toward an attitude of gratefulness. If I can take ownership of the gifts of God, can I not take ownership in the miracles of God? When this happens then all things become possible with His involvement. A positive and grateful attitude then becomes essential to my health, to the relationships around me and, most importantly, to the ability of God to play a part in my life. It is the bedrock of unleashing the gifts of God in our lives and the foundation of empowering our faith.

Now that I have built this foundation of understanding, I want to point out that at the top of the list of tools at my disposal lies Faith. Faith is something which is so easy to wrap our minds around, yet so fleeting at times. Faith has been described aptly as believing in the evidence of things not yet seen (Hebrews 11:1). While I understand the intent of this description, I somehow feel the general understanding and interpretation of it falls short of the true meaning. Faith, for me, is something more than just believing, and it is not always reliant on evidence. If we require evidence for everything we believe in, we live in a very narrow understanding of God's influence in our lives.

I believe this is the first and a somewhat superficial level of understanding and describing faith.

In a book entitled *What Would Jesus Do?* written in 1950 by Glenn Clark, there is a story of a small child who was included in a prayer for healing. As the prayers were lifted to God, the child focused intently on the words but, most importantly, although it was not written, you got the feeling that she simply imagined the outcome as being complete. There was no doubt in her mind; she simply knew it was done. When the prayer was over, she arose and skipped out of the room stating "There, it's done!" To have that youthful innocence to believe it is done is something we all strive for, but there is something deeper here. The understanding that when she said Amen, she didn't believe it was so, she knew it was so. This is the level of faith that God wants us to have. To move our faith from believing to knowing, removes all doubt and empowers the miracles of God. This is the level of faith I desire and confess. An absolute faith where I no longer believe, I simply know.

The appointment time with the doctor came and we entered his office with our tools intact. As he entered the room, we were simply waiting for the confirmation of what we already knew. Our urologist is a matter-of-fact type of guy. In his profession this serves him well, and it is comforting to have someone who deals with the facts in these situations. As he read the findings, we quietly absorbed the information. "The results of the biopsy came back and the two things that we were looking to find out were whether or not you have cancer and, if so, is it aggressive or not. Your results indicate that of the ten biopsies taken, five (or half) of them were positive. This confirms that you have prostate cancer. The second part of the test, to determine aggressiveness, is rated on a Gleason Scale of 2 to 10. Yours came back at 7s and 8s. To summarize, this indicates that you have an aggressive form of prostate cancer."

We were expecting the news to come back as cancer, but the inclusion of the word "aggressive" became unsettling. As we discussed the remaining information, we made plans for additional tests to determine if the cancer had spread outside of the prostate. Only when this test comes back will a path of treatment be able to be established. Leaving the appointment with another appointment and further tests scheduled, we were again placed in the waiting game. As noted earlier, I really don't like this game, but we were learning to play it well. We had become trapped in the medical loop. The only thing we could do was to stay focused on the tools we could control.

We went home and spent the rest of the day contemplating the meaning of it all. As the level of seriousness increases, so does the level of stress. This became evident when my sister Judy came over to discuss the results later in the day. As we sat outside on the lanai and laid out the newest information, emotions came to the surface. Marilyn's tender heart overflowed, and you could tell she was becoming overwhelmed when the tears came forward. It was during that conversation that Judy asked me a question that made me contemplate something I hadn't thought much of before. She asked, "Are you afraid?" I stated, "No I am not, but I am concerned!" I truly was not afraid.

For me the concept of being afraid or having fear, comes from the unknown. This indicates a lack of knowledge or experience about a place, condition, or problem. The control of fear then lies in seeking out the wisdom and experience necessary to understand the challenge. I knew that this is something in my control and while I currently did not possess all the information, I could obtain it. The other component of this comes again from faith. As mentioned before, I have already been shown the outcome in a series of dreams and knew the destination. The unknown was still part of the journey, but I have been on a journey all my life. This is just another detour we must take.

The reality is that I was scared. Being scared is not the same as having fear. Scared has its origins more in facing the unknown and not fearing it. To say that I am not concerned about the situation is not true. This is the most serious challenge Marilyn and I had ever faced, but we faced it together—with God and our relationship there to comfort and direct.

The key for me lay in the controlling of my mind and the doubts that occasionally flair up. My prayer for this journey then became "God, help me in my unbelief and transform my faith from belief to knowing. You are a good and gracious God, and I pray that You will use my life for Your glory. Lord I pray that Your healing hand will be on my mind, body, and soul, and that You will deliver us through this bumpy road in such a way that everyone will know that You are God. Bring us peace and understanding in Your methods and words of praise from our mouths; in Jesus' Name. Amen."

The tests that we scheduled when we left the office were both scans. These are designed to help determine if the cancer has metastasized outside of the prostate. The first was a CT scan, which looks for the evidence of cancer in lymph nodes in the pelvic area. If the cancer has in fact moved outside of the prostate, it will most likely find its way into the nodes. Next, was a nuclear bone scan, which looks for evidence of abnormal activity in the bones— other places this cancer will typically move to outside the prostate.

These tests are in fact not definitive, as it is possible that they return no evidence or slight evidence, and neither are conclusive. They were, though, the most credible methods currently in play at that time, and we pursued them.

The day of the tests arrived and, with the waiting over, we headed to the imaging lab. The bone scan involves a two-step process. First, you receive an injection of a low-level radioactive substance, which will eventually find its way into the bone. Once you have been given the injection, you have to wait three to six hours before the scan. The body will immediately begin processing this and removing it from your system. This means that to assist in its removal you are required to drink an excessive amount of water, which leads to going to the bathroom a lot.

Oh, by the way, your urine during this time is also radioactive so you need to be careful and wash your hands frequently. With all this effort the one thing that I found disappointing was the fact that I did not acquire any superpowers like they do in the comics, although I did tell my son, Josh, that I had. I exclaimed to him that I was now Batman. His response by text was uplifting and humorous and provided us a source of conversation for the remainder of the wait.

After receiving the injection, we were released from the facility to go about our day for the next three hours. We had some errands to run and basically just killed time, keeping in mind that we needed to stay close to a restroom to get rid of all the water I was drinking. We eventually made our way back to the lab where the rest of the tests would be performed.

For individuals who are going through these types of events in their lives, it is important for those around them to provide an environment of support. Facing the unknown for all is a scary situation, but when it is personal it can become overwhelming. The staff and lab technicians at the imaging facility were excellent. Even during the injection portion of the test there was a conscious attempt to keep me informed and to answer questions. Fear arises from the unknown, knowing provides comfort.

We were ushered through the facility to the CT scan area where Marilyn was instructed to sit in the waiting room, as it was not healthy for her to be in the room when they were doing the scan. I was taken to the CT scanner where, after removing all metal objects, I was instructed to lay on the carrier. The scan was simple and quick. It only took around seven minutes from start to finish, and we were escorted to the nuclear medicine wing. There, the lab technician took over and instructed me to again get on the carrier and let him do all the work. Marilyn was given a chair and, after he noticed her shivering, was given a warm blanket. The machine raised, inserted, and tracked me out of the scanner. The entire process was scheduled for a 45-minute window but after reviewing the first images, he determined that no further scans were necessary.

Not knowing how to take that comment, we took it as a positive. After all, it could have meant that things are normal or that there is no use looking any further because the evidence is there. His words were comforting when he stated, "There is no reason to look any closer at any area because they all looked clean to me." This was followed by the ever present "But I am not the interpreter." He had been doing this for 39 years and one could assume that after seeing literally tens of thousands of these images, he would have an educated knowledge albeit not the final say.

We left the imaging lab that afternoon with copies of the images on a CD and a hope of good things beginning to emerge. Still, we had to wait for the interpretation and meeting with the doctor to determine the next steps. We decided that we were going to build on this momentum and take the weekend off from the worry and concern. The weather in west coast Florida is absolutely beautiful. Looking out at the sunshine, palm trees, and lush greenery just makes you feel good. Stepping out on a late October day into 80 degree temperature seems to melt away concerns. This we did and enjoyed the weekend with each other.

Next, came the first appointment with our new family physician. Upon entering the room, having filled out all the required forms and having had vitals taken by the nurse, we introduced ourselves. My first question to her was "Are you ready to go on a journey with us?" She smiled and said, "There is a story behind that and we will see." She then began the process of becoming familiar with us as new patients and, as the conditions unfolded, you could sense compassion in her comments. This, coupled with her acute knowledge in the medical field, gave us both a peaceful feeling. Completing the exam and having discussed her take on the conditions and acquiring a review of the medical services and offices in the area, we left knowing this would be a good relationship.

We returned to the imaging lab to confirm that the CD's we had been given indeed had images on them. When viewed, they appeared to be blank, unformatted discs with nothing on them. Realizing that the medical industry has their own software, we were unsure. The lab staff were again very gracious and rescanned the discs and confirmed that the images were in fact there. This time they also included printed copies of the professional opinions rendered from the readings. These opinions are made by trained specialists whose job is to analyze the images and look for evidence of the disease outside of the organ in question. To our surprise and delight, both reports indicated the scans were "grossly normal."

While we welcomed this information, we knew that the final view and opinion would be left in the hands of the urologist. However, we both knew that the true meaning behind these results was confirmation of God's presence and works in my life. Eagerly waiting for the report from the urologist, we went to our morning appointment the next day to confirm what we already knew. The doctor, as I mentioned before, is a no nonsense kind of guy and, as he reported the findings, he was cautious to warn that just because the images were negative, he felt that because of the statistical probabilities, I still had cancer which had spread outside of the prostate. While I appreciated his skills and abilities, I reserved his opinion as that of a medical professional whose life, existence, and decisions are based on statistical outcomes. Both Marilyn and I knew that this was only one component of the journey and that he was only one of the tools we were applying to the problem. The other tools, including Faith, do not bow to statistical analysis and, therefore, cannot be quantified. Yet these are the ones we place our trust in and follow the evidence of.

When I reference tools, I must share a story to provide perspective. As the doctor was providing his diagnosis, he attempted to provide some words of encouragement. "Mr. Fuller, there is good news. With all of the advancements in technology through new drugs, refined radiation, and better understanding of the cancer you have, we have the ability to add months to your life."

I simply turned to him and stated, "Whenever I am faced with a challenge, let's say an electrical problem in my home, I go to my garage and pull out my electrical tool bag. I will then take that tool bag to the problem and fix whatever is broken. If it is a plumbing problem, I will grab my plumbing tool bag. If it is a carpentry problem, I will grab my carpentry tool bag. When you come to my problem, cancer, you bring your tool bag. It is full of tools such as your experience, your training, and advances in technology and medicines. With this tool bag in hand, your assessment is that you will be able to add months to my life.

You and your tools are important to me and I will use them. However, they are not the only tool bags available to me. I have one called Faith, one called relationship, one called attitude, and others. In many cases, these are more powerful than yours. If it is all the same to you, I will use your tool bag along with mine and see you in twenty years." He simply looked at me, paused for a moment, and responded, "Okay," before he went back to his mechanical routine.

Having discussed the possible courses of treatment, we decided that the most prudent course of action would be to set up an appointment with a radiation oncologist who would ultimately become a part of our team but, more importantly, would be able to provide a second look at the data to assist us with making choices in the path toward a cure.

There are five possible treatments that are typically used to treat prostate cancer. Then there are combinations of these, which expand the options exponentially. The challenge is to discern the information and sort out the path that best fits you and your goals and expectations. Each of these have benefits, complications, and results to review. It was lucky for us that we had been researching these prior to the appointment and had acquired a basic understanding of the treatments before we arrived.

Not being in denial but rather in an informed understanding that God would do His part, we simply did ours. After doing our research and receiving the urologist's input, the path that felt most in line with our goals was to have a prostatectomy, completely removing the prostate. After a four to six week healing time and a three-month waiting time, we would monitor the PSA levels to determine the success of the surgery. If, in fact, all of the cancer has been removed the levels would drop significantly to manageable levels. This would most likely be followed up with external beam radiation to ensure that any possible cancerous cells outside, near the prostate are also destroyed. Again, this would require a three month wait after the initial surgery plus the monitoring time before radiation could begin. In addition, before the surgery, I was going to receive Lupron hormone blocking therapy, which would inhibit the growth of any cancerous cells that may have metastasized outside of the prostate.

Leaving this doctor's office, we drove to the next doctor's office that had connections with a premier cancer institute in our area that had been highly recommended to us. It would give us the added benefit of being partnered with them. To begin a course of action with this in our back pocket again felt right. Blindly walking into the office, we were able to set up our initial appointment with the radiation oncologist for the following day. Home again, we continued the wait, thankful that with each passing day, a clearer picture was emerging.

During our down time, we found that there are two possible courses of action. The first is to transform oneself into a research ninja, completely immersing our entire existence into the wealth of unorganized and, in some cases, meaningless information available when doing research on the web, consuming day after day of time. We have found that before we embark on this cyber space journey, it is wise to prepare ourselves by dropping to our knees and praying for patience and discernment. While the information gained is important in assisting to make accurate and informed decisions, the reality is we may have just passed up on the one true opportunity to affect your health in the process. While we are there on our knees, praying, we should be asking for God's hand to be present in our lives, in the lives of those who are a part of our treatment process, and in the healing. This reminds me of the story of someone who is looking for something when all the time it is by their side. So many times in my life, I have looked to the external, whether for knowledge, wealth, love, or friendships, when they were standing by my side or living inside me all the time. Learning to recognize the treasures we already have has been something I have been working on and, in reality, has led to the most rewarding payoffs.

The second course of action is to completely ignore the situation. While this can be the easiest solution, it does have a component of irresponsibility to it. To be able to completely remove yourself from the problem and ignore its inevitability is to shirk responsibility for your own life. This, as I mentioned, is the defeatist attitude that I dare not allow in my life. The real solution lies somewhere between these two extremes. Somewhere, between ignoring it completely and having the challenge totally consume you, exists a balance where peace can exist. I must be careful to seek this place in order to maintain my own sanity. This place is where I can be approached by others and affected by God's will while continuing to prepare myself for future decisions. Sometimes, I think this is the hardest thing we need to do, to seek balance.

When we first started this journey, it was like we had been immersed into a murder mystery. As you are entering the room of life, you suddenly find out that someone has been killed in that room and the killer is still there. As soon as that news is revealed, the room immediately fills with a dense fog. You can and will be overwhelmed by the sense of helplessness that floods over your body. You face forward motionless, wondering what just happened while quietly in your spirit reaching back for the doorknob so you can simply exit the room to safety and claim a "do-over." The doorknob does not exist. There is no reverse strategy in life, only a forward path. As you stand there, the fog begins to thin slightly, allowing a somewhat clearer picture of the room to appear. As we continue to peel back the layers of the unknown, we are in fact wiping the mist off our glasses while the fog evaporates.

The challenge we faced when we were first told I had prostate cancer was no longer the same challenge we faced that day. The cancer had not changed but we had. We were more educated; we had enlisted others on our journey; we had accepted our responsibility toward its cure, and had surrendered the outcome to God. Slowly, the fog was being removed.

The following day, as we entered into the office for our next scheduled visit, we were becoming more prepared. Armed with our growing knowledge, we met with the radiation oncologist who had been recommended to us. He was very pleasant and well informed. He reviewed my reports, all the while keeping us updated, as his actions overflowed into the conversation. Next, he performed his own examination. I don't want to say that you ever get used to it, but the process was becoming way too familiar. After the exam, we entered a conversation regarding his thoughts toward my condition and a course of action.

47

While not completely in conflict with the urologist's opinion, he did provide additional insight into the paths of treatment. His diagnosis remained true to the previous diagnosis. Interestingly enough, again, the facts remained the facts. His recommendation for treatment was slightly different, which he substantiated with statistical studies and data.

Every person is created unique by God and, therefore, responds differently to treatments. That being said, there are basic biological functions that remain true and, therefore, a level of confidence can be derived through repetitive results. This is where the statistical data enters into the picture. Based on personal and statistical results, the radiation oncologist felt that the correct course of treatment would be to follow the path of hormone blocking therapy, brachytherapy (which is placing radioactive "seeds" into the prostate), and then follow up with external beam radiation therapy. This path has proven over time to give the best results and was his recommendation. He encouraged us to take some time, but not too much, to think it over and let him know when we were ready to start treatment.

As we were seeking information, several sources had brought up the afore mentioned Cancer Center to which the radiation oncologist had connections. This facility is a premier cancer research and treatment center affiliated with a university and only 25 miles from our house. Taking cues from the various recommendations, we began doing additional research into this organization. Their website indicated that they have a very credible patient library where information can be gathered in the presence of trained medical staff. Again, with the intentions of continuing my understanding, I preregistered as a patient to gain access to the information. After the appointment with our radiation oncologist, whose office was in a small town quite a ways north of us, we decided to drive to the Cancer Center library, albeit quite a ways out of our way, and do a little research. The facility is impressive. It is an entire medical hospital dedicated to the cure of cancer. We entered the library from the parking lot through a back entrance where we gathered information and chatted with the staff. They offer new patient and visitor orientation presentations, and we happened to be there when one was starting. The presentation was very informative and opened our eyes to the offerings they provided.

After leaving the Cancer Hospital, we journeyed home. During this time Marilyn and I, as usual, were having a discussion about our thoughts. She was strongly suggesting that I make an appointment with one of the Cancer Center's medical oncologists to get a second opinion. My thought process has been, and continues to be, to focus on identifying the issue, which we had done, to seek out paths of treatment, which we had done, to find partners we were comfortable with to assist us, which we had done, and to move forward. The idea of going down those paths again just didn't make sense to me. My response then became "Why?"

This difference of opinion led to an evening of anxiety, which neither of us needed or enjoyed. During this time, our conversations turned to the need for her to find a support organization and system which can help her through the journey. In all honesty, I had become so focused on my journey that I forgot for a while that we were on this trip together.

After coming to some sort of understanding on the issue and sleeping on it, I woke up the next morning and called the Cancer Center to schedule an appointment. They offer a wholistic approach to cancer care. They not only treat the patient but also treat the family and friends of the patient. Cancer is a horrific disease. Because of the emotional attachment we have and the ambiguity of the disease, it spreads to those around us, typically not physically but definitely emotionally. They have developed programs that treat the emotional spread of the disease by involving, caring for, and supporting those around a cancer patient. This is the support that Marilyn needed and expected. While it was not all encompassing, it was beneficial and welcomed. Later that day, they called and set up an appointment with a medical oncologist who would be responsible for the total care program. We were to meet with him on Monday, so we again had to wait and continue to enjoy life.

We had intentionally been very selective in choosing the individuals we included in this process, not because we were ashamed, afraid, or trying to protect anything, but more for our own self-preservation. We are blessed to have a multitude of friends and family who would immediately become our support group and walk the journey with us. The challenge is in the communication. Because they are all close and dear to us, we were becoming more and more compelled to keep them informed in the process. While this would open up the support channels, it would require a significant amount of time and would distract us from the task at hand, which was to identify, educate, evaluate, and chart a course of action. While we were dealing with all of this, we knew that taking on the additional challenge of including and informing others would be too overwhelming.

As we had been peeling back the layers and clearing the fog, we had not been extending our communication borders. I can't tell you how much this played a part in our ability to cope with the problem. To live my life as an entirely open book would be an impossibility for me. I could not handle the constant demands that this would require. It is no wonder that famous people burn out early or turn to other methods of escape. Their emotional being is drained on a daily basis and there is no recharge time.

Another challenge was to manage misinformation. Sometimes a person, loving though they might be, will take what they know and attempt to fill in the unknowns, which leads to uninformed false conclusions. This inevitably leads to a wrong set of information being shared. We have all played the telephone game when we were children and know how funny it can be. The challenge is when you are dealing with real problems and emotions it, moves from comedy to tragedy quickly. This process of limiting who we informed also allowed us to bring our friends and loved ones into the fold with a personal touch. They are our friends and family for a reason and deserve this.

Chapter 3

Sharing and Deciding

Now that the picture was becoming more clear, I decided it was time to include my work colleagues into the circle. One of the major concerns I had was to not inundate our son Josh. Because he works closely with and for the same company, he could potentially become collateral damage when the questions and support start flowing. To help counter this, we began the process of talking with him about what other's responses may be and to empower him to control his space. He must be able to draw his own boundaries and allow himself to say "No" if he needs the space to recharge and process.

Also, I had drawn on my employer's experience who had gone down this path before. Because it is a family-owned business, he had to deal with this type of thing way too many times. So, through his example and counsel, I put out a corporate-wide letter that informed of the situation, the methods of support, and a promise of future updates.

The response was what we hoped for. The company Marilyn and I work for is full of compassionate and caring people. Their return emails were words of acknowledgement and support, which were amazingly uplifting. They are, in fact, my family, and at times it caused me a certain level of pain to not always be able to include them in the process. But we were still peeling back the layers of the solution and required private processing time for our own peace and sanity, so I know it was the correct decision. To our friends who may read this, I want you to know that your love and friendship was not in any way less important than those who were included earlier in the involvement. It was simply a method of controlling our ability to cope. You all matter to us and we care deeply for each of you.

This same process has been something we continued to do with our non-work friends and family. Holding our hand cautiously on the throttle, we were reaching out and informing those around us only little by little. To date, we have been able to remain in control of our emotional state, not to say that there were not times when we stumbled, everyone does, but more that we have been able to keep interactions minimal for our own health.

Another important component of this informative stage lies in the ability to draw on the experience of others. Seeking to grasp onto what the journey was going to be like, we searched for others who had gone before us. What we found was a limited amount of information concerning the stories of those brave souls. Most of my circle of friends tend to be conservative in nature. This proud, conservative attitude is more evidenced in what they don't do as opposed to what they do. They don't expect anyone to do anything for them. They typically face their challenges head on and take sole responsibility for them. They don't brag about their successes or complain about their failures. They typically walk their life out quietly, in dignity and peace, accepting their circumstances and worrying more about others than they do about themselves. This translates into stories never told and challenges faced without many knowing. Only when pressed, and if they feel it will encourage or uplift someone who is facing a similar obstacle, will they reluctantly share. These revelations are typically followed by our inevitable response, "I didn't know."

I can definitely relate to these people, as I have very similar tendencies. To those who have opened up, I will say thank you for sharing, relating, and encouraging on a personal level. Still, there are countless numbers of people who need to hear your stories. As we searched for people to relate to, we found their voices eerily silent. The challenge with this is that it becomes easy to interpret this as an absence of positive results and, therefore, the opposite is assumed, meaning failure. This is a challenge for those whose support system has not been established. They could easily become overwhelmed with the matter-of-fact methods of the medical community and their statistical data, dropping into a state of depression. Stories need to be told! Recognizing and connecting with others who have walked the path is an essential part of remaining focused on the destination of cure. While I respect your desire to stay out of the limelight, I encourage you to step out and share. It can be a priceless gift of hope that someone is desperately searching for.

Monday we began the day with the anticipation of meeting with a medical oncologist at the premier Cancer Center. Our hopes were that enlisting a cancer specialist who would be able to look at the challenge confronting us at a higher level would bring some clarity to the process. The drive to the center is normally a somewhat relaxed 25-mile trip, as it had been when we visited their library the week before. This takes between 35 to 90 minutes depending on the time of day and traffic patterns. One thing about living in populous areas is you can always count on the traffic. Most of the time it is manageable, and the fact that we are in a slower and supposedly more relaxed place in our lives, we simply plan ahead and enjoy the ride. This day was a good day and the trip allowed us sufficient time to stop to get some lunch.

Arriving at the center, it was a blessing to have complimentary valet parking available for patients at the majestic, welcoming front entrance. While they whisked our car away to the parking garage, we made our way to the appropriate department where we began my registration. What happened next should have provided an advanced clue on how this visit was going to play out. Sitting down and after working through the unexpected news that our appointment had been cancelled, we filled out the paperwork and then managed to work through the scheduling issue and get a new appointment with the doctor, without the need to leave and come back. After a brief wait in the waiting room, we were escorted to the common area where I was weighed, tested, and asked the usual medical questions. We were then led down the hall to our assigned consultation room.

The medical oncologist entered and began the interview/analysis phase. As we were going over my condition, we were interrupted when his pager went off for the second time. After excusing himself, he exited with the instructions that he would return in around five minutes. During this break, I needed to use the restroom, so I seized the opportunity. Of course it was occupied, so I patiently waited for the occupant to finish. An elderly lady exited and while I was moving out of her way, another gal came down the hall and entered. Still waiting patiently on my turn, I again should have realized the theme that was presenting itself. The second gal eventually exited and exclaimed, "Were you waiting for the restroom?" and before I could respond, she turned and walked away. She had no clue, nor did she care about the answer, as she made her way back down the hall.

Finishing, I returned to our room where I found the doctor had returned. He was attempting to show something to Marilyn on the computer when it went dead. They were trying to resurrect it to no avail. He decided that it would be best if we moved to another room where we could continue our appointment with the technology he required. Marilyn left for her turn in the restroom. He returned and exclaimed, "I have found another room, come on" and abruptly walked back out.

I gathered up the records we had brought with us, entered the hall and found him nowhere. Not wanting to randomly open doors, searching for our new location, I must have looked confused enough that one of the nurses asked me what I needed. Claiming that I had lost my doctor, she helped me relocate him in the new room. Entering and getting settled, I expected him to wait for Marilyn to return before beginning but soon realized he was unaware she was not with me. Marilyn now, upon exiting the restroom, was faced with the same dilemma of not knowing where to go. Eventually finding us, she joined the already ongoing interview.

Using a marker to circle the test results a couple of times, he proceeded to take us on a new journey all to itself. He talked about the various paths of treatment, including the risks and benefits of each. The challenge came when we attempted to make sense out of any of it. Many of you have been left scratching your head when you've innocently picked up one of those information brochures that come with a prescription. Well, imagine doing this with a live person who is regurgitating the facts of five different medications. We looked at each other, shrugged our shoulders, and both immediately realized that the gift of relating and communicating to others is not universal. Some people have acquired it, some are attempting to acquire it, while others don't even know it exists. We happened to be sitting with one who fit into the last category.

While we both understood that he had an extremely good grasp on the medical aspects of prostate cancer, he was not capable of communicating any of this to us in a language we could understand. When you are facing decisions that have significant impact on your quality and quantity of life, the two things you are looking for are clear and concise information and someone who can confidently travel with you on your journey. We found neither of these in the doctor in front of us. After spending almost an hour again circling the information he was attempting to communicate and handing us a paper with his inadequately explained recommendation, we finally realized that our chosen path of treatment was correct for me and that our original doctors were the correct ones for us. While our expectations of the appointment did not pan out, the end result left us with a sense of confidence about our chosen path. I guess it all works out in the end, even if the process isn't what you expected.

Because of our experience at the Cancer Center, we lost confidence in them and their services, we never went back. Marilyn found the support she needed elsewhere: some through the resources we discovered at the Cancer Center and some in the literature and pamphlets available at our local oncologist's office. Remember, Marilyn is a research ninja. She was ever seeking out information and guidance on the web. A word of caution, though, to those who choose this path, you will need a strong level of faith and discernment to navigate these waters to know what to hang onto and what to throw out. She also gained strength through our church family, who was an ever constant source of support.

Leaving the campus, we decided to initiate the process of setting the treatment plan into action. We would forego the prostatectomy surgery. We called the radiation oncologist to set up the first hormone blocking injection. He informed us that we would not need to see the him at this time and would begin the scheduling process for the brachytherapy surgery of inserting the radioactive "seeds" into the prostate. We were feeling a level of relief because we were finally entering into a new phase toward the cure.

Beginning the exiting of the information phase, we were moving into the action phase. Even though we understood that this phase will have greater hurdles and challenges, it was definitely welcomed. We were transitioning from the unknown to the known, albeit with an understanding that there would be new unknowns and new difficult experiences we would need to face.

Now that we had defined a plan and set it in motion, we decided to open up the channels of information even further. We began the process of notifying the next level of family and friends. Surprisingly, it became an easy process. When you are armed with a greater level of information and a path to travel, the questions and responses become predictable. This leads to a level of confidence that is comforting to all. Each step in the process was affirming our belief in the cure and removing the questions and doubts from our minds. This is exactly where I needed to be, fully committed to the process, knowledgeable of the pitfalls, and moving confidently toward the cure, without doubt.

The process of setting up the treatments proved to be more of a challenge than we expected. With the ever-increasing demands on the medical professions, the simple tasks of setting appointments and carrying them out became burdensome. Couple this with the knowledge that we already possessed a path to a cure, it can lead to elevated stress in what should be a time of comfort and peace. We called the office of the radiation oncologist and were placed into a voicemail system. We left a message, indicating our intentions to begin the therapy and then patiently waited for the phone to ring. One, two, four hours went by and no call materialized. We called back only to leave an additional voicemail message. By this time, it was late in the day, so we resolved ourselves that the call would come in the morning.

The next morning, we still had no call. It appeared our only option was what had worked the last time, to just show up at the office. We entered and made our way to the front desk. The receptionist, with whom we had already made a connection, smiled when she greeted us. After explaining that we were attempting to set up an appointment to begin treatment, she informed us that she was already working on it and was waiting for the insurance approval, which seemed to be a major hold up. To accelerate the process, we went ahead and scheduled an appointment, informing the scheduler that we needed to speak to the radiation oncologist at the same time (since he wouldn't be the one giving the injections), which we could eventually cancel if needed. Leaving the office, we were pleased to be back on the forward moving track.

Chapter 4

Action

When the scheduled appointment came, we waited patiently, no pun intended, for the nurse to escort us to the exam room. While I was not anxious about beginning this new series with its side effects, it was the next step in the journey. It was about 40 minutes after our scheduled appointment time when they finally escorted us to the room. There, the nurse did the usual check-in stuff while informing us about the procedure of the injection. When we expressed interest in speaking with the doctor as we had requested when we set up the appointment, she looked at us funny and exclaimed, "That wasn't on the schedule." She was great and, sensing our concern, left the room to attempt to herd the doctor our way. After reentering, she instructed that the injection was going to be administered in the buttocks and that I should drop my drawers, turn my toes inward to reduce the strain and bend over the table. Lupron, the hormone deprivation agent selected, is administered as a deep muscle tissue injection. This requires the needle to be sufficiently long to reach those deep tissues. You've seen cartoons where the nurse enters the room with a syringe with a three-foot needle attached to it and the patient faints. Now, it wasn't that big, but it did cause me to take a second look. Once my shocked, bulging eyes shrunk back to normal, she carefully inserted the needle and administered the dose.

The doctor entered the room and amazingly took the time to answer our questions about the frequency of injections, the time frame for the brachytherapy, and the run-up tests needed before the procedure. He did what every patient desires and expects from their physician. He sat down, took the time to review the reports, answered our questions, and inform the nurse of the next path of action—all of this without a "scheduled" appointment. We left with an affirmation that we had definitely made the correct decision. I can't overstate how important it is to have a working relationship with your caregivers. This doctor went the extra mile and it went a long way to provide comfort and peace.

We still wondered about the opinion written by the medical oncologist at the Cancer Center. His recommendation was to enhance the Lupron injection with an oral supplement of bicalutamide. This combination acts as a total blockade of testosterone in the body, effectively providing the equivalent of chemical castration. This is a radical approach, but, with the high PSA levels present in my body, he felt it would provide the best results. After reviewing this information with the radiation oncology, he agreed but warned that the side effects, although low risk, would be more intense with this approach. Although I was not looking forward to the hot flashes, they would be a welcome reminder that the drugs were working.

The side effects of the injection were evidenced soon after we left the office. Because of the deep muscle penetration, the surrounding muscle tissue quickly became sore. The level of pain continued to increase over the next two days. It was tolerable but did remind me that the journey had begun. After the third day, the pain level began dropping to a dull ache and eventually disappeared. A few days later, there was little evidence of the actual injection and life had returned to a form of normality.

Next, was an appointment with our general practitioner to bring her up to date with our chosen path and progress. She digested the information with interest and, after reviewing the reports which had been forwarded to her, agreed that we were on the correct path, at least for us. This was followed the next day with a visit to the urologist where we began, as he would be the surgeon who would be performing the brachytherapy procedure, while the oncologist would actually insert the radiation "seeds." These are tiny pencil lead like pieces of highly radioactive material that are inserted into the prostate gland.

The urologist again reminded us about the challenges we were facing, and instructed us to begin setting up the next series of tests and appointments. This included a procedure called a volume study which he described as a glorified ultrasound test during which they completely map the prostate. It is done at the local hospital under IV sedation. This "map" is then given to the radiation oncoloogist who works with a radiation physicist in mapping out the placement and quantity of seeds needed. They then order the materials and have them delivered to the hospital, awaiting the procedure.

The challenge with this was the coordination of all the offices involved. We were now working with the urologist, the radiation oncoloogist, The ultrasound technician, the hospital, and the anesthesiologist to perform one simple test. To this end and with an accelerated timeline, driven by us, we were again mired in the waiting game. What again seemed like a simple thing to accomplish actually involved extensive coordination of personnel and offices.

In addition to all of this, the urologist will also perform a cystoscopy. This is where they inspect the urethra and bladder for any unusual formations or conditions that may lead to complications during and after the seeding. This is a preventative procedure that reduces the risk of complications. What you don't want is to be faced with additional intrusions into the treated area after the treatment, as it will have a greater risk of failure. So, to that end, we were again scheduling something else.

In the middle of all of this was the realization that we had agreed to spend Thanksgiving week with Marilyn's cousin and family in Pawley's Island, South Carolina. Their daughter is our Goddaughter who, along with her husband and children, have become very dear to us. The thought of not being able to fulfill the promise was saddening; however, the urgency of my condition as presented made the decision easy. Stress creeps into your life in many ways. I have learned that the true source of stress is being forced to do something that violates your core beliefs or convictions. To not be able to spend time with people you love and promised to be with is most definitely a source of stress by this definition.

The volume study was scheduled on the day we were to leave for South Carolina, of course. Understanding the difficulty of scheduling the urologist, hospital, and surgeon together within the time frame needed to allow us to continue the accelerated treatment plan, we decided to have the procedure done and then leave for the seven-hour drive. We were not on a strict timeline to get to our destination, so, if needed, we would stop and rest or spend the night. The plans were then made and the family notified. The morning of the study arrived, and we were all prepared. We had packed our bags for the trip, loaded them into the car, and planned the trip ahead of time.

The night before the procedure was prep time. Anyone who has had the opportunity to prep for a colonoscopy understands the procedure. The only thing that afforded some level of comfort was that I had experienced this before and therefore knew the process. While it is not one of the most pleasant memories in my life, it was manageable. Waking up early in the morning, with me fully cleaned out, we headed to the hospital.

We arrived at the outpatient surgery prep waiting room, checked in, and proceeded to wait for my turn. The staff was wonderful. Soon, I was moved to the prep area where the nurse team began getting me ready for the study. Along with the volume study, they were also going to perform the cystoscopy to determine if the urethra was clean and unobstructed. With the inclusion of any obstructions, the seeding operation would face greater complications. I fully understood the desire and need to perform this procedure; however, in the back of my mind, I could imagine them sitting in a room saying, "While he is sedated, I can think of another orifice we can send a probe down." I know this is not the case and that they were simply staging the ultimate surgery for success, but I couldn't help letting that passing thought play out.

During the prep time, the conversation with the nurses soon made its way to what to expect after the procedure. Instructions included taking pain medication, not straining, and getting plenty of rest. When I informed them that we were leaving for a trip immediately, they literally stopped what they were doing and, like animated heads, both turned to face me in silence. After a moment, the primary nurse simply shook her head and said that was probably not the smartest decision I had ever made. I assured her that we would be careful, take our time, rest when required, and that Marilyn had graciously volunteered to drive, as I would be on medication. Soon I was prepped, the urologist came in to review the procedure, answer any questions, and we headed off to the surgery room.

The surgery event was nothing for me. I was placed in "la-la land" and woke up forty-five minutes later in the recovery room. There, I was gently brought back into the world of the coherent and given liquids to rehydrate. I felt great and could not understand why they thought that travel would be a bad idea. In reality, what did I know? After all, I was on pain medication and could not feel a thing. When I was sufficiently recovered, it was down to the car, off to home for some final preparations, and then on our way to celebrate Thanksgiving.

The trip was uneventful. With Marilyn driving, of course, we took our time on the way up the coast. We stopped and stretched, got something to eat, and reloaded me with the pain meds to insure a comfortable ride. There was an uncomfortable feeling, but nothing unmanageable. We arrived at a large house with seven bedrooms, full of loving family, where we nestled in for an evening of conversation. The next morning, I was off the pain killers completely and life was back to normal. We thoroughly enjoyed our stay and celebrated Thanksgiving being truly thankful for the lives we shared. The walks on the beach were wonderful and only hindered by the fatigue effects of the Lupron injections and bicalutimide pills.

The brachytherapy (radiation seeding) was scheduled for two weeks after we returned. During that time, the radiation oncologist and the urologist reviewed the results of the volume study and formulated a coverage map for the seeding. This involved accurate measurements of the prostate, accurate radiation exposure calculations, and accurate patterns of insertion. While all of this was going on, we were confidently optimistic that the procedure would bring us closer to the ultimate goal of "cured." As discussed above, the outcome was never in doubt. I/we knew that the end game was I would have a tattoo. Still, the anticipation of the process can lead to concern or ultimately to anxiety if allowed to fester in your mind.

I can see how people may get wrapped up in the emotions of cancer. I suppose this is not a fair statement, as an emotion can be attached to any traumatic event. Anything that causes you to become aware of or question your mortality will play games in your mind. Only a firm conviction of a positive outcome can guide you through the roller coaster ride. I was fortunate to have the stabilizing knowledge of the destination, which God had revealed in a dream early on. Never did I doubt the wisdom He shared nor question the outcome. I cannot explain the peace that flowed over me. It was simply there.

Marilyn on the other hand did occasionally have a slide backwards. She was amazing and, although her fear stayed mostly subdued, I could tell there was concern. Sometimes I think it is harder to watch a loved one go through the valley than to walk there yourself.

The day of the seeding arrived and, again with prep work the night before, which was becoming all too familiar, we headed off to the hospital. Once we arrived, the process became familiar and automatic. Check in at the surgical desk, quietly wait to be called, remove your clothes, put on the gown, answer questions, hold still for the IV insertion, answer questions, wait, join small talk, answer questions, wait, endure more small talk, wait, and then go. I hope that I never need to get used to this.

Because of our understanding that the outcome was already predetermined, the stress associated with the procedure was not present. However, the mere fact that you are about to be put under and have radioactive substances inserted up your rectum and into your prostate where they would remain, can bring thoughts of anxiety to even the strongest souls.

Next, I was rolled down the halls to the operating room where a team of nurses and doctors were waiting. After shifting me onto the operating table, the staff went about their duties with a comforting efficiency. Next on the agenda was the familiar "What is your name and what are we doing?" question followed by a very brief "See you in the post-op" response and then lights out.

The beauty of modern medicine is in the ability to place the patient into an unconscious state during surgical procedures. Typically, there is an inclusion of an amnesia-inducing drug in the IV. This is present because, as good as the anesthesiologists are, they place you in a fine line state of unconsciousness, but occasionally that line gets crossed briefly, and your senses begin to re-awaken. During those brief moments of discomfort, the drug keeps you from remembering any of it and, therefore, if it does not exist in your memory, it never happened. The next thing I remembered was the calm voices and sounds around me as I slowly woke from a dreamless rest.

Lying there under the warm blankets, attempting to regain a sense of me, I had a peaceful feeling. My mind was simply re-awakening to the life ahead. Full of pain medication and resting comfortably gave a false sense of effortlessness to the procedure I had just experienced. At that moment, my thoughts were, "This was a piece of cake, what was all the fuss about? I feel fine." What a false sense of reality. When the full force of the elimination of the pain medication became real, I fully understood what really happened.

The doctor came in and briefed us and was very happy with the procedure. He walked us through the whole process, indicating that they had inserted 82 seeds into the prostate in the desired and mapped pattern. They experienced no complications during the surgery and fully expected recovery to proceed normally. These are the words you want to hear from a surgeon after surgery, and they only served to reinforce our understanding that the outcome was predetermined.

But wait, what is this tube hanging out of me, and what about the bag on the end of it? Having the process explained to you during the pre-op overview and experiencing the aftermath are two totally separate activities. Yes, they did explain that there would be a catheter inserted which would remain for several days to prevent any swelling from blocking the urethra. However, to actually have it hanging out of me was not what I had pictured. I suddenly understood what it was like to be a puppy tied to a leash, but at least the puppy was tethered at the neck. Me, not so much. When I was sufficiently alert and mobile, it was over to a wheelchair where I would be transported to our car and then, ultimately, home.

Marilyn was such an angel during this process. I could not imagine going through this, or any procedure, without her Love and care. She was truly a blessing and, although I was attempting to be a perfect patient, we all know that I did have those moments. She, however, simply took it in stride, and we emerged albeit a little bruised but mostly unscathed. I do Love her more than I sometimes let her know and am truly thankful that God allowed one of His best to be a part of my life.

At home, we had a few days of muddling through the inconveniences of catheter living. A home nurse was assigned to me and made her first visit to verify that all was well. She ran the usual tests to determine how I was coping post-op and provided us a contact number for any questions or emergencies that may arise. Then it was sleep in the chair, get up to go drain the catheter bag, back to the chair. Eat, drink, sit, and drain. I did not get used to the spasms from the catheter. With the urine flow pretty much guaranteed, the actual need to relieve myself was not required; however, occasionally there would be a spasm which caused severe pain and a false sense of urgency. At one time when the spasms were strong, I was moving toward the bathroom when I leaked around the catheter. I was on a strong antibacterial medication that caused my urine to be bright yellow. We found out that it is also a permanent dye. Eventually the stain came out of the carpet, but it served as a reminder of the procedure.

After three days, the nurse came and removed the catheter. I have always been able to find the humor in most circumstances. However, standing with your drawers down with a woman holding onto a tube hanging out of your penis and trying to not imagine the worst while she is saying, "This won't hurt much" was one of those times when I truly struggled to stay positive. In hindsight, it was funny and, she was correct, it didn't hurt much and was over quickly. I guess this is the same process that animals go through when they are castrated. The relief of the pressure was instantaneous and welcome. The burning sensation when urinating was minor and went away quickly. All had returned to a sense of normality, even though I was aware there were radioactive substances inside me, killing selectively for my own well-being.

Life returned to the closest thing to normal we had experienced in a while. The effects of the Lupron were ever present. Tiredness, fatigue, hot flashes, and tenderness had become a part of my new normal. Naps were almost always a part of my day. I would get up in the morning, log on to the computer and do whatever work I could muster. My place of employment was remarkable and sensitive to the struggles I was facing. They would pass off limited tasks that had few deadlines and allowed me to complete them at will. There was an element of stress associated with this, as I have always attempted to give more than expected or received. This process of getting more than I was giving was foreign to me and uncomfortable. I felt something was out of balance and that I needed to contribute more. I learned a life lesson during that time, which is "the giving spirit exists in all individuals." Sometimes you are the giver and sometimes you are the recipient. In all cases, it is always a blessing and I am truly blessed to have such a caring group of family, friends, and co-workers.

Next on the agenda was the external beam radiation. The urologist's part in this journey had come to a holding place, and now it was time for the oncologist to take over. His specialty was in radiation oncology, and he and his team would be administering the radiation treatments. The seeds were working inside of me, killing the targeted cancer cells. They have a 90-day half-life in which there is nothing else to do but wait while they deteriorate and perform their silent killing mission.

During this time, we managed to stay somewhat active, taking walks, doing minor exercises, and mostly reflecting on where we had been and where we were going. It was also when we began the prep work for the external radiation. This involved CT scans to determine the radiation sequence and duration. The initial CT scan was to determine a baseline, map the targeted radiation paths, and determine the radiation dosage that would be required to treat the surrounding area. Targeted properly, radiation is an amazing tool for good. Targeted poorly, it is a tool of destruction. The goal is to target the radiation into cancer-confirmed or cancer-suspected areas and to minimize the effects to surrounding organs and tissue.

As a part of the preparations, I received my first official tattoos. They were three small reference dots placed on me to serve as permanent markers for alignment. Lasers were used to align the markers that would ensure I was always positioned the same on the table. This allowed for accurate targeting of the radiation beams to the specific areas. They were also markers used for future procedures. Since the paths chosen for the radiation beams will have become sensitized, any future attempt to radiate cannot cross the paths of those beams. If they do, collateral damage will result in the killing of healthy tissue.

Next were the leg molds, which were formed out of urethane foam. As I lay on the table, they injected liquid foam into control bags that conformed to every nuance of my legs. This allowed for stabilization of my lower body during my upcoming radiation treatments. After the casts were made and the scans completed, I was allowed to re-dress. Sometimes the simplest process ends up delivering the greatest result. With the image of full circle radiation soon to be beamed through my body, it was comforting to know accuracy was utmost on their minds.

Radiation treatments would not start for four more weeks. Again, we were placed into the holding pattern where faith is allowed to blossom. I don't know any other way to put this. Your mind will dwell on whatever you choose to feed it. Occasionally, I would get the urge to feel sorry for myself and begin to doubt the potential outcome. Immediately, and I mean in the blink of an eye,

I would catch that thought and dismiss it from my very being. There was no room for doubt and faith to exist together. Having been shown the end of the journey, I simply refused to entertain those thoughts.

We enjoyed Christmas and New Year celebrations with friends. During the wait period, we had had no other assignment except to allow the radiation to do its deed, so we managed to soak in the holiday season. Funny how the little things become more important when you are facing life challenges. Visiting with friends, celebrating in their parties, and enjoying family all seemed a little sweeter. We sometimes pushed the limits on my energy levels, but there was a possibility that we may not get to do those things again. For now, our goal was to live life. Finally, in February, the day arrived for radiation to begin.

Someone once told me that peace comes from within. While I do believe that our destiny is within our decisions, I also believe that outside influences greatly affect how we arrive at those decisions. The staff at the oncology office were excellent to work with. Their assurance and mannerisms only served to maintain a confidence in the decisions we made to journey down this particular path. During the first scheduled appointment, we discussed the treatment plan, process, and potential side effects before entering into the radiation room. The staff introduced themselves as though they were privileged to be able to deliver their specialized service. I can only make the comparison of walking into a favorite restaurant where the owner is truly grateful that you are there and fully understands that you could have selected other places to dine. The expectation, therefore, is to deliver a service that is deserving of your trust in the establishment.

Asked to disrobe and put on the gown, I was instructed to wait in the small waiting area. Others who were going on their own journey were present, quietly sitting for their turn. I cannot resist the opportunity to engage others, especially when the stakes are high. Sometimes the simplest comment can make the most difference in the obstacles we face. Not knowing if I was going to be blessed or to bless, I would reach out to my fellow travelers. "Hi, what are you battling" would in most cases lead to an abbreviated conversation. Some were one or two minutes depending on our appointment times, while others would last a while. Some, like I, were beginning their journey and others were coming to the end of this chapter. Nonetheless, we all had something in common, the restoration of life and normality.

My turn came and I was escorted into a room where a large machine graced the center. Many of you have either had CT scans or seen CT scan machines. This tool consists of a floating table which positions you precisely inside a rotating ring where an imaging or radiation device is directed to traverse your being. As it rotates, there are whirring and clunking sounds which are the only indications that something is actually being done. Your job is to lay perfectly still while the technician directs the machine to do its job. Now you fully understand the importance of the leg molds and the alignment tattoos. Briefly, a great appreciation for technology rises up along with the appreciation for those who had gone before you and their sacrifices to get where we are today.

Seven minutes. That's all it took to deliver the levels of radiation required for my treatment plan. I was helped onto the table. The molds were placed on my legs, the technician pressed controls that manipulated me into an approximate position, then he or she left the room. Lying there in the mostly vacant room with instructions, "DON'T MOVE," my options were limited. Trying to glance around the room, I realized the device itself was about all I could see. Slight glances beyond the formidable ring, I could make out the sources of the three lasers that were targeted at me. Their ultimate destinations were the tattoo dots gifted to me during the preliminary planning phase. I could easily have drifted off into dream land if given enough time. It was uncannily peaceful, with only the faint sounds of conversations well beyond my perception.

This silence was broken when the technician announced over a speaker near me that the process was to begin. Suddenly, the table began to move up and down, twisting and tilting all at the same time. While the movements were subtle, they were perceptible and too complex to be controlled manually. Technology was again making itself apparent in a physical way, as I realized there was a computer controlling the movements, driven by sensors with the precision of perfection.

As soon as the motion stopped, there was a desire to sit up and see if, in fact, the lasers were on target. This urge was dissipated by the knowledge that I could never see this. Any movement would change the positioning and jeopardize the accuracy of the radiation beams. So again, lie still and trust that all is well.

Quiet returned to the room only briefly. Very soon, the ring again started making sounds and moving, carrying its head around my body. Whirring and humming, it made its journey full circle. Next, a brief quiet again followed by now softer and gentler motions of the table. The lasers position the exterior body in an exact position and the first pass was a CT scan that looked at the inside. Based on the initial scan during the planning phase, the computer now took the level of positioning to a much higher level. It was now positioning my tumors and internal organs back to an image mimicking the initial scan. This image was what the radiation team used to determine the targeting sequences, allowing the maximum impact on cancer cells, while minimizing the impact of its deadly force on healthy portions of the target path. All I could think of was "WOW" and be thankful for the people who have chosen to seek the knowledge to design, understand, and operate this technology.

Next, the ring returned to life, circling my body. The sounds were different this time. It's hard to describe the differences, but they were different sounds. The part of the head that drove the imaging passes remained silent, and now the radiation delivering components were active. In place of the constant sounds as it moved, I could hear intensity rising and falling, starting and stopping sounds, all while the head slowed and increased in speed. The radiation was being delivered to its intended target. It was avoiding sensitive organs and tissue, taking clear paths through open tissue, intensifying because the angle to the prostate was buried deep through the hip, and softening as it passed over the groin area—all this with the goal of delivering a measured dose to a specific target to facilitate cancer eradication. Seven minutes from the start of the process, the technician returned to the room, manipulated the table to allow me to exit the machine, removed the molds, and helped me up. Being led back to the waiting/changing room, I was instructed to get dressed, and told, "See you tomorrow."

Twenty-five times this would be repeated. Monday through Friday, always at the same time, 8:20 in the morning. The interesting thing for me was I felt no indications that any treatment was being delivered. Some experience pain, some nausea, some become anemic, while others have rectal issues. I was only experiencing a slight decrease in energy levels. This was hard to distinguish between the latent effects of the seeding and the Lupron.

At this point, fatigue was a normal state for me. God had already delivered to me the most precious gift which was knowledge. The knowledge of the outcome was all I needed. I was on a journey, traveling through unknown and unexperienced events, but I knew the end of this part of the story. This allowed me to focus on the journey and not get caught up in the fear and doubt most experience.

As I mentioned before, the time in the waiting room was an opportunity to share in this experience. One person in the room with me was a gentleman from the islands. He would sit, quietly awaiting his turn, mostly in the end corner chair. I would sit down, sometimes close to him, and ask, "How are you doing?"

He would simply respond in a definite island slang, "Hanging in there, mon."

To that I would encourage him to simply do that, as it was apparent from his mannerisms he did not want to engage in further conversation.

On one occasion, after several shared visits and a repeat of the same conversation with the "hanging in there" response, I felt compelled to respond differently. I turned toward him more pronounced than previous encounters and said, "Wow, that is amazing. I would like you to picture what you are saying. To simply hang in there implies that you are holding on to the rung of a ladder. Your feet do not have a rung to step on to take away some of the stress, so you are forced to simply hold on for dear life. Over time your arms grow tired and eventually fail, and all you have managed to do is wear yourself out. This is not a place you or I would ever want to be."

To this he responded, "Then what would you have me do, mon?"

My response was simply, "Climb or let go. Do not just hang in there."

He quietly stared at me and asked, "What would you have me say, mon."

I replied, "Simply tell yourself you are getting better every day." At the end of that comment, I was called to my appointment. Getting up to leave, I smiled and nodded as I left the room.

After that conversation, I did not see him again. He was not at the next scheduled treatment day. As I approached the end of my treatment regiment, this gentleman had no longer been in the waiting room. For several days, I would go and see others, but island man was not there. I hoped that his treatments were over and that all was well with his condition. But, still, the last conversation we had loomed in the back of my mind.

On my final day of treatment, a celebration was planned. This is not an unusual event as the treatment center always celebrates the end of a treatment regiment, with the honored tradition of ringing the bell. On that day, near the end of March, I entered the waiting room where a more than usual number of men were sitting, waiting for their appointments. Turns out that there had been an issue with the computer system, which required the technicians to completely reboot it to clear the errors. To my surprise, the island man was sitting in his usual spot.

As I changed into the gown and chose a seat a few chairs away from him, I asked again, "How are you doing today?"

His response was both refreshing and encouraging. He said, "Getting better every day, Mon!"

"That's awesome," I replied.

He went on to explain, "A while back there was a man who told me to stop hanging in there and to climb or let go." He decided to stop staying where he was and begin climbing toward his cure. I mentioned to him that I was so happy for him. He looked at me more carefully now and exclaimed, "It was you, mon. Thank you!" It was my time to share at that last meeting, and I felt both happy and honored that God had used me to reach out to someone who was in need of His love. The technician called my name and off I went to my last treatment, blessed that someone who was suffering was displaying rays of hope.

The final treatment was one which was celebrated by both the patient and staff at the clinic. The process was quite simple. When you exited the treatment room, there was a bell hanging on the wall, which you rang with all the enthusiasm you could muster. As it rang through the halls, everyone in earshot would cheer and applaud, sharing in your accomplishment. When the congratulations had subsided, the staff would present you with a certificate of completion to commemorate the occasion. Then, unceremoniously you would dress, grab your certificate, and head home.

Chapter 5

Evidence of Success

As August approached, with all treatments over, except for one more Lupron shot, there was nothing to do physically. Our lives were returning to a form of normality and, without the scheduled appointments looming over our daily activities, we could finally focus on the reality of living in Florida. While sitting on our patio, I immersed myself into paying more attention to and thoroughly enjoying the warm weather with the palm trees overlooking the golf course.

Even though there was never a doubt about the outcome, there seemed to be a sense of relief that this chapter in our lives was coming to an end. Never do I want to take what we had gone through for granted or without appreciation. God's presence has intensified in my life. Flowers smell sweeter, gentle breezes seem more welcome, words kinder, and joy closer because of the path we have traveled. I had made a promise to myself that the tattoo would become a reality once the outcome was confirmed.

Now with the goal in sight, we would need to wait for the test results, which were scheduled every six months. As discussed above, the Lupron would mask the true PSA readings and should not be trusted in determining an actual level. They were, however, important because an elevated level in the presence of Lupron would indicate a severe abnormality. So, we would go to the office, have blood drawn, and wait for the results. A few days later the results would be presented. "Undetectable, less than 0.9%" were welcoming reports from the oncologist.

One year after that last Lupron injection, the drug had purged from my system. No longer was there anything that could interfere with the actual PSA test results. Whatever the true levels were in my body, they were about to be revealed in the next test. Off to the office, blood drawn, sent to the lab, and home to wait. Three days later the follow-up appointment for the true PSA results was one to remember. Again, the statement "undetectable" was read, and the assurance I had from the beginning that I would be cured was now confirmed to the world.

All my self-imposed obstacles to getting the tattoo were now removed. There was only one thing left to do! On November 1, 2016, I proudly sat in a chair, with my wife looking on, and had the word, that our faith had been hanging onto, tattooed on my right shoulder. After all the years of talking people out of tattoos, I was ready to show the world the symbol of my journey and to openly confirm to all who will listen, "I am a cancer SURVIVOR, and let me tell you how God helped me through the valley."

After receiving the tattoo, I have had several opportunities to share the story of how it came to pass. As a cancer survivor, I have become more aware of people's needs. It is interesting that the word "cancer" now often enters my conversations when before my journey, it rarely did. Sometimes it is introduced by others and sometimes by me. In any case, the opportunity to share my tattoo story and the hope which came along with it has materialized. Somehow, sharing the story before the tattoo seemed a little less impactful. Now whenever I share it, the question of "Did you get it?" is always asked. Pulling up my sleeve, revealing the word "Survivor" leads people to a sense of peace. I know that faith brought me to this point, and I am sustained by it. Having the evidence of past faith is reassuring.

PHASE II

THE NEW JOURNEY:

NEW DISCOVERIES

MORE INFORMATION

MORE ACTION

Chapter 6

Meet the World's Best!

Having a history of prostate cancer dictates that one should remain vigilant. While the treatment strategies we had undertaken, along with our faith, had produced remarkable results, we were fully aware that our lives continue. This demands that we keep a watchful eye on any potential threats that may arise. Based on our desires and the doctor's recommendations, we had continued with 3-month screenings of my PSA levels. While we knew in our hearts that the treatment was successful, we also understood that we should be aware of any indications of recurrence. But based on the previous test results, we were transitioning our cycles to a 6-month testing of PSA levels, which happened to coincide with the blood tests our family doctor had ordered.

While I don't mind needles being stuck into me, as I mentioned before, I do not think of them as a source of pleasure. If I can reduce the number of times I will be someone's pin cushion, then sign me up. We discussed including the PSA tests with our normal blood tests with our oncologist, and he agreed it would be a good move, with the condition that he be copied in on the results for his review.

With our newfound confidence and our lives returned to our new normal, we were beginning to enjoy the magnitude of our decision to move to Florida. For those who aspire to someday move toward semi or full retirement in a place where snow is celebrated somewhere else by someone else, I can only say, "This is amazing."

We have been blessed with having family close by. This, coupled with the ability to travel for both pleasure and work back to our northern Indiana roots, makes is doubly delightful. Add to that a new set of great friends to complement our lives in Florida and we have the perfect balance. The full repercussions of our original decision to move were finally coming to fruition. For those who have not experienced "GREEN WINTERS," I highly recommend them.

My midpoint routine blood work was done with the inclusion of the PSA tests for the first time. The routine went as usual: go to the office, sit in a chair, get poked and drawn, and leave for the day's activities. All went as planned until the following day's phone call from the doctor's nurse. "Mr. Fuller, can you please give me a call when you get a chance?" was the message left on my voicemail.

History has shown that this normally does not bide well for me. A simple "Hey, Mr. Fuller, the results are back, and all is well" would have been much more comforting, but still no alarms should go off yet. My return call was met with the words, "Everything looks good, but your PSA level has climbed to 1.9, over one point higher since your last test in January. You should have your urologist check into this." This in itself would not have been a cause for alarm, but the fact that it came after the treatment process to achieve complete and proven annihilation of the cancer was. Our sure-fire regiment was now showing a chink in its armor.

This led to the possibility of doubt to creep into our thoughts and that was concerning. Still, nothing to worry about. We must follow the rabbit down its hole to see where it leads and not jump to conclusions. Next on the list: set up an appointment with the urologist. We scheduled the appointment and took the records with us to the meeting. The doctor's practice must have been thriving. He had built a new facility and, during our absence, had moved his practice into this nice new building. Nothing was familiar, yet this was all too familiar. The routine was and is, sign in, pee in the cup, wait, move to the exam room, answer questions, wait, and then the doctor comes in.

As you may remember from a previous chapter, this guy is our auto mechanic personality guy. His no-nonsense, get to the facts, and move on approach was welcome at times. This was one of those times. "Mr. Fuller, I have reviewed your PSA levels and found they are indeed climbing. As you know, in your case," he continued on. I'm not attempting to provide dictation here. You get the drift. His summary was direct and to the point. Facts: Your PSA is climbing, you were at high risk with your original diagnosis, your prostate has been effectively killed by the treatment administered and should not be producing any antigens. The Prostate-Specific Antigens must be coming from sources outside of the prostate. The recurrence of prostate cancer after treatment is upwards of 50%, follow-up treatments are minimal, but we can put you back on Lupron and wait and see what happens.

As we are now fully aware, Lupron suppresses hormones which in turn inhibits the growth of cancer cells that thrive on hormones. It is a functional tool used in the management of prostate cancer. It is like this: imagine you get up one morning and go out to your garage and find there is a small puddle of antifreeze under your car. Realizing this is not natural, you go to the store where a clerk tells you that there is this miracle product that you can use to fix it. "You simply dump some of this 'StopLeak' into the radiator and, voila', the leak disappears," and he is correct. The problem is you have not actually fixed the problem. Your radiator could be corroding from the inside gradually, and over time it will fail in a catastrophic event. Lupron is sort of like that. While effectively lowering the PSA levels in your body, which indicates the cancer is shrinking or going away, it is, in fact, just stopping the cancer growth for a while. Now will that bandage hold for the duration of your expected end of life? No one knows!

Discussing the possible courses of action, we determined it would be appropriate to redo the original nuclear bone and CT scans, and use them as a baseline for this new adventure. He warned us that the PSA levels indicate that any potential growth sites may be too small to detect at this time and to not get our hopes up. Isn't it funny that some people never get it? Life without hope is not worth living. If I were to ever settle into a sense of hopelessness, I would give up on life itself. That state of being does not resonate with me or my faith at all.

Remember the toolbox analogy referenced earlier? Right then and there, we decided that we were going to use his toolbox. Not for what it contained but more for where it could take us. Next on the agenda: schedule the scans, set appointment with oncologist, begin looking for a new urologist, and dive into research, again. After we had a chance to do some more research, process the information, and understand where this may lead, we reached out to our son and let him know what was going on. His reaction was as expected: cautious, concerned, and optimistic—at least outwardly. We reassured him that all will be well and that we will keep him informed.

During our previous experience with the imaging center, I had exclaimed to him that after being injected with radioactive isotopes, I had somehow become Batman. Since that time, I have come to the understanding that Batman was never affected by a radiation source to create his super persona, so therefore I could not have made that transformation. However, on one of our trips up north, we were at Josh's house (where we normally stay) one evening, and he pulled up the movie, *Deadpool*, on Netflix. Deadpool was a character in a comic book who was exposed to excessive amounts of radiation which caused him to develop super human characteristics. Now, here is a guy who fits into my mold, albeit absent my spiritual component. So, this time I proclaimed to Josh that I expect to be transformed into that character, and Josh's response was priceless, "You'll definitely have more fun!" We laughed, thought about it for a moment, and moved on. Enough said!

Again, the regiment was all too familiar: go in for an injection, drink lots of water to flush it through your system and out of your bladder, return in two hours, pee, lie down, scan, pee, lie down, scan, pee, get dressed, pee,

95

pick up the CDs, pee, and leave. Okay, maybe I went a little overboard on the drink lots of water thing. But I do take instructions seriously and, on this journey of eliminating cancer from my body, I did not want to have anything inside of me that could potentially be carcinogenic for any length of time longer than necessary.

The meeting with our radiation oncologist went well. We picked up the results of the scans and took them with us to the appointment. Reviewing the documents and his records, he concluded that there is something going on, and we should be diligent in pursuing a course of action. His recommendation of going on Lupron was also taken with a grain of salt but with a higher level of confidence than when the option was delivered by our urologist. The difference, interestingly enough, comes not from their levels of knowledge. Both are equally knowledgeable and skilled in their professions. It comes from the level of compassion and caring with which they share. The feeling of caring goes a long way in building and maintaining trust. Trust is the key component to a relationship that allows people to interact with each other and effect change.

He also suggested that we perform a sodium fluoride PET scan to assist in determining where the cancer may be hiding. These tests are much more detailed, allowing the treatment teams to develop more specific targets of treatment if possible. Also, we agreed that it would be prudent to retest the PSA levels to eliminate the possibility of false readings and/or lab differences. So blood was drawn and sent off to the lab for evaluation. Leaving the office, we committed to re-educating ourselves on prostate cancer and, more specifically, the recurrence of prostate cancer.

Home to process, we now had a task ahead of us: to find out all we could on the testing capabilities and new technologies afforded to prostate cancer patients and caregivers. Marilyn has long been an avid researcher. She thrives on the details and, to some degree, enjoys the hunt. It is in her very nature to seek out information, almost as though she is shopping, which she thoroughly enjoys.

I heard it said once that men are hunters and women are gatherers. Men, when hungry, will venture out into the wilderness, see a prey, kill it, and eat it. Then the hunger has subsided.

Women will take on this same challenge as a journey. They will venture out and begin collecting different berries and herbs. They will take an assessment of the wildlife present and then formulate a dinner plan using all of the most desirable components available to them. Finally, they will prepare a meal worthy of a king, fresh with the assortment of options available to them. Both methodologies accomplish the same end goal. Neither is right or wrong and, when blended, bring harmony to the process. I love and respect her ability to gather and share, especially in times like these. She brings a component to the table, which I sometimes overlook.

During our down time, if there was such a thing, we both immersed ourselves in fact finding. Her path led her to advanced imaging capabilities for the detection of recurrent prostate cancer. Again, the challenge is defining where it hides in your body to be able to effectively treat it.

Two potential techniques seemed to rise above the rest, with one of those shining to us like a beacon in the night. Mayo Clinic in Rochester, Minnesota had developed

97

a PET scan that uses Choline C-11 isotope as the tracer for detecting cancer in soft tissue and bone. The technique uses the need of prostate cancer cells to have choline during the rapid division process. So the cells perform a rapid uptake of the radioactive choline C-11 isotope, into their structure. This allows the PET scan to accurately detect and pinpoint the locations of prostate cancer cells, even at low concentration levels. The challenge is the C-11 isotope has a 20-minute half-life and must be produced in a particle accelerator close to the patient. This leaves one primary location where the test can be performed: Mayo Clinic, Rochester, Minnesota.

We contacted our radiation oncologist and shared the insight we had found. He informed us that the PSA scan came back from the lab and it had in fact climbed another point, sitting at 2.9 now. We agreed that now is the time to move forward with whatever our chosen path is. His remarks led us to believe he was and still is the correct partner for our new journey. "That test is advanced and if you are willing to pursue it, how can I assist?" Again, I cannot overemphasize the importance of having individuals around you whose desire is to affect a cure on your behalf. They are truly looking out for your best interest and not worried if they are benefitting from the process. "I will write a referral to Mayo for the testing, if required" was his comment in our parting conversation.

We reached out to Mayo the following morning and found their caring touch comforting. After a brief explanation of our situation, we were referred to an admissions person who began the process of defining what and who would be most effective for our relationship with them. She gathered the facts, asked appropriate questions, noted our concerns, and determined that Dr. Eugene Kwon would be the best fit for our initial review.

Dr. Kwon is, in fact, the doctor who was instrumental in the development of the C-11 PET scan process in the United States. He is arguably one of the best prostate doctors in the world. Our thoughts that we are going to bring onto our team someone of this caliber was extremely comforting. This was also followed by the thought that they must think my condition warrants someone who is the best in the world. AAAAGH! Knowing that we were going to "the guy" affirmed our decision to contact them.

The lady on the phone also confirmed that once a patient has begun a regiment of Lupron, the C-11 scans cannot be performed. It inhibits the flow of the tracer into the cancer cells and renders the scan results useless. We understand that there is strong evidence to support the use of Lupron as a tool to slow or shrink the cancer growth, but it is equally important to accurately determine where cancer cells exists to facilitate a cure. A new sense of urgency was being interjected into the process. We ended the initial contact with instructions to mail or fax my medical records to them for their review. This was great, we were moving forward with positive action.

To ensure we were providing Mayo with the most accurate information, we reached out to the three primary contributors to our medical journey. Our urologist, our family doctor, and our radiation oncologist. Explaining what the reasoning was for obtaining the records and the urgency, we were greeted with three very different responses. The urology staff informed us that there is a charge of $1.00 per page for them to provide us with the records and that they have up to 30 days to generate them. The family care staff also informed us that there is a fee for generating the records, and once they had determined the cost, and we paid the fee, they would print the documents for our retrieval. The oncologist staff said, "Come and get them." Each had properly defined their priorities and helped to reinforce our decision to keep, or discard and replace, the members of our new team. It appeared that we were now looking for a new family care doctor as well. After paying, prodding, and otherwise being an annoyance, we received the records, assembled them, and faxed them to Mayo. Now the wait began again, but with the knowledge that we are attacking the issue with all of our might and, most importantly, with our faith wide open.

If we have learned anything on this journey, the most important lesson would be that you must be your own advocate. The concept of being vested in the process simply states that we have the most to lose if failure were allowed to rear its ugly head. Therefore, the individuals who must take the lead in seeking out a cure to our cancer, is us. This concept of personal responsibility escapes many. I have met and been around people in my life who simply allow the "professionals" to determine the courses of action or, even worse, to simply sit back and exclaim, "God will deliver and if not, it is His will."

To those I say, "When did you remove yourself from the responsibility of living your life?"

God wanting us to surrender our lives to Him is not an admission of helplessness. It is the recognition of a partnership where we agree to be an active participant in the process and allow Him to simply be our leader—to keep Him in our thoughts and lives and not to exclude His love and direction. This is, in fact, the true sign of a healthy relationship, not one based on independence or codependence but rather on interdependence.

To that end, we have been actively pursuing information, direction, and knowledge. God has blessed many on this earth with wisdom and compassion toward the sick. Their passions have driven them toward finding cures to even the most complex diseases and illnesses. They have brought great progress to mankind and saved (health wise) millions of people from suffering and loss. Some individuals believe that this is doing the will of man and not allowing God's will to prevail. But I say that allowing these advancements to take an active role in our quest is simply the responsible and faithful thing to do.

This reminds me of the story of an elderly man who placed his faith in God when the flood waters began to rise around his home. He exclaimed "God, deliver me from this threat" and went about waiting on the porch. As the waters rose, a truck of rescuers approached and asked him to get in with them. His reply was that he was confident God would deliver him and that he had and will continue to trust in Him. The waters continued to rise, and he had moved to the second floor when a boat approached with the same request. His response was again the same as before. Next, he climbed onto the roof as the waters rose higher yet. Soon a helicopter flew overhead and lowered a line to lift him from his peril. Again, the response was returned, "I trust in the Lord to save me, but thanks and Godspeed." Soon the man was swept off the house and perished. Upon arriving at the pearly gates, the man asked Saint Peter, "Why weren't my prayers answered?" Saint Peter exclaimed, "We sent you a truck, a boat, and a helicopter. What more did you want?" I believe that God delivers answers to prayers many times through men. Sometimes these men acknowledge their participation in this process and His involvement; other times not. None the less, God's hand is in the process, and if we always keep our relationship with Him in focus, we will see it, even if they don't.

Providing Mayo with the appropriate information had become a bit of a chore. It seemed that our sense of urgency did not match others'. Not a surprise; however, it did become a reality check and a reminder that this is our journey. They happen to be spectators and occasional contributors to the process. Marilyn was a ninja in her pursuit for order. I mentioned earlier that her world has an amazing sense of structure unlike mine. This demands that the ducks in her life behave. So, to manage the order, attitude, and appearance of her ducks requires her to delve into more information and structure.

Neither of us were having restful nights. One or both of us remained up in the wee hours, unable to sleep. Unfortunately, it almost never happened at the same time. One night it was me; the next night her. Consequently, we were both tired and not usually on the same schedule. For me, naps became more precious. There never seemed to be an appropriate time to take one, but sometimes it meant the difference between functioning or not.

So, six months after I had gotten the "SURVIVOR" tattoo, we had the initial appointments at Mayo for preliminary evaluations set for the first of May. Along with the C-11 PET scan, there was an MRI and bloodwork scheduled. However, the scanner for the desired C-11 scan was not available until the first of July, so all tests were re-scheduled. This delay for the scan appointment was concerning to both of us. With the possibility of using Lupron as an inhibitor still imminent, and being dependent on getting the scan done first, it simply meant we would be in this dreaded waiting game again. With the knowledge that the cancer is most likely growing at an accelerated rate, any delay simply meant more treatment and more cancer.

We had inquired about moving up the scan appointment due to a cancellation or/and if we could go onto a waiting list. The demands on the scanner come from various departments and, therefore, they were not informed of the cancellations. It would be best advised to call them and request they check availability. Knowing this would be a moment-by-moment condition, I asked if I could call every hour. Thankfully for them, the response was no, and that the appropriate time frame would be around every two to three days. I said thank you because we did understand that you need to step away from the issue periodically, otherwise you will be consumed mentally long before the cancer kills you.

After a couple of days, we contacted Mayo about assisting them in acquiring the pathology slides from the original biopsies from the original lab, and, during that call, I asked if there were any openings due to cancellations. After a few minutes, she returned and announced she had moved my appointment up about 45 days to just 8 days after the initial appointment. The timing was perfect.

Mayo then reached out to the pathology lab in Florida and had the slides sent for their evaluation.

Time is required for the pre-certification process to ensure the procedures are covered by insurance. The C-11 Choline PET scans are very expensive, and the inclusion of insurance's involvement is extremely comforting. If there were questions or information required to support the authorization, we hoped eight days would be sufficient time to seek out and provide the answers. Patience and faithfulness. This is what is required for God's hand to become visible in the process. We continued to be vigilant and trust in the outcome.

As we continued to explore the paths of treatment for recurrent prostate cancer, there were two very distinct paths that presented themselves. The first and most prevalent is palliative care or simplified, placing a bandage on the "ouchy," and waiting for it to potentially heal. This is also sometimes called symptomatic treatment. The challenge with this type of care is that, by definition, it does not address the true issue. By masking the problem, the hope is that the body will heal itself and the problem will just fade away. Cancer does not work like that, and individuals who opt for this plan of treatment are just kicking the can down the road. Eventually, statistically, the cancer will return and, hopefully, there will be newly created palliative treatments available. This will allow you to continue to kick the can until you have reached what your expected life span would be. Then, you would die from some other cause and become one of those statistics who died with prostate cancer and not from it.

The other treatment plan is curative treatment. This is where you and your team set out on a journey to eliminate the cancer from your system once and for all. This requires the proper and precise identification of where it exists. Once this has been identified, treatments can be designed for complete eradication. Seeking out individuals and teams who truly are actively seeking curative treatment options, for us, was and is critical to ending at our desired goal of cure and maintaining our mental health and attitude. The challenge with this path will be at what cost? Financial and time commitments are much greater on this path. Individuals in the medical field who embark on this journey with their patients are becoming high-demand people. As more patients are becoming informed of the alternate paths toward treatment, the more these individuals and teams are sought out and employed. The time commitment comes from that personal responsibility thing. It is and always has been our responsibility for our care. Ronald Reagan, when dealing with the dissolution of the Soviet Union's nuclear arsenal made the statement of policy to "Trust but Verify." This is wise advice for everyone who is on a medical odyssey.

Along this journey, I had somewhere and at sometime made a transition in thought toward spirituality. I have always been drawn toward an understanding that God is a personal God. The idea of having any person or organization insert themselves in the middle of our relationship was totally foreign to me. Years ago, I shared with a colleague that I had a selfish prayer. While others would pray and actively pursue moving closer to God, I would pray that He would come closer to me. I believe that I have a purpose here on this earth and that I should be fully engaged in building relationships, comforting, and mentoring others along their spiritual journey. The idea of moving closer to God implied that I must move away from where I am at, albeit mentally. It says in James 4:8 and implies in Jeremiah 29:12, "Draw near to God and He will draw near to you." I had already, years ago, drawn near to Him. I was asking for the phase of Him drawing near to me. Most importantly, I needed God to be with me daily, hourly, even continuously. With this mindset, I would need His presence with me always and, therefore, be reminded of our unbroken relationship.

During this journey, I have relied heavily on His presence and the friendship we share. I speak to God not just as a worshiper, but as though He is a partner, a counselor, and teacher. Do not get me wrong, I do not in any way imply that I am equal to God. What I do confess is that I am in Him and that He is in me. We are in fact inseparable. A part of His spirit was surrendered to my care while I take every breath. When the last breath has escaped from my lungs, this shared piece of Him will return to His eternal presence. My challenge here is to not exclude Him, or ignore His presence, or allow life to interfere with our bond. By thinking, acting, and walking with Him every moment of the day, I truly know that we are connected and inseparable. This walk through cancer has been an interesting test of my faith. I am thankful for our relationship and the comfort only a friend can bring. Prayers become more like conversations. One thing that makes a solid, healthy relationship is that both parties are good listeners. In mine with God, He listens and I listen.

Answers come to me in God's language, which includes feelings, thoughts, nudges, and acts of Love from others. Through this conversation, my understanding grows. We will move through this and emerge together, immersed in our strengthened relationship.

Chapter 7

The Best Answers

The anticipation of the trip to Minnesota now became the focal point of our lives. Not the all-consuming type, but rather the feeling you get when you are about to get on a roller coaster for the first time. You know that it will be okay and that you will be safe, but your energy inside wants to come out. We did not allow it to consume us, as there were preparatory things that needed to be done before our trip north. We, after all, did not know how long this trip was going to last. Would Mayo want additional testing, begin treatment immediately, treat us there, or allow us to go back to Florida? So many unanswered questions only meant that we should prepare for several scenarios simultaneously.

We quickly realized that we considered ourselves still in control and that we had not fully released the challenge to the companionship of God and trust Him for the outcome. The chaos eventually subsided to a dull roar and then to a routine.

We had our flights booked, hotel arrangements made, were satisfied with our research to this point, and had an opportunity to accept well wishes from other friends and family, including some surprising ones. An unexpected visit from our nephew and his family from Germany served as a welcomed distraction. We received them with open arms, and would have loved to spend more time with them, but, sadly, our pressing responsibilities wouldn't allow it.

A little while later, some dear friends of ours had pre-planned a cruise, which would pass them through our area for a couple of days. We had to adjust our schedules a little but had time to have dinner with them and get caught up.

Sometimes, as you get consumed in these journeys, you feel as though you are alone in a wilderness. It is moments like these which pull you back to an understanding that you are only on a journey alone if you choose to be. Including others, at the appropriate times, is one of the most comforting things you can do.

We are creatures of relationships and our sense of loneliness arises from keeping loved ones at arm's length. By allowing them to come closer, the journey seems less formidable. After saying our goodbyes to family, our friends took us to the airport on their way to their cruise—both of us heading out on a voyage with anxiousness and anticipation.

We arrived at our destination late that evening and were shuttled to the hotel by an on-call cab. Once there and checked in, the bed was a welcome sight. We settled in and had a chance to catch a warm cookie at the front desk to calm ourselves before we returned to our room and drifted off to sleep. I mention the cookie because there are certain childhood memories we all share that trigger a sense of comfort. Sublimely, these items or events help to soothe over the stress we feel or deny. They take us back to a place in our lives when everything seemed alright—where the world felt warmer and the skies seemed bluer. Cookies are that trigger for me. When I was a young boy, we would come in from a hard day of playing and seeking adventure to find that Mom was baking a fresh batch of chocolate chip cookies. Hurrying to get cleaned up, we would manage to make it back to the kitchen in time to take the cookies off of the cookie sheet as soon as they were cool enough to handle. The anticipation of warm chocolate cookies along with a cold glass of milk was almost unbearable as the smell drifted through the house. I still associate this with the love Mom had for us.

Somehow, this sense of returning becomes a source of comfort. Healing is a lot like this. Whenever we face a sickness or challenge to our health, we simply desire to return to that place where we started. To go back or to reset our lives where all seemed well. We need the understanding that, as we are seeking a cure to the cancer in front of us, we are not seeking to go to a new or foreign place, but rather to return to what we already know and have experienced. We need to return to that place of wholeness from whence we came—that place where God placed us in the beginning.

We spent the following day, Sunday, relaxing by the indoor pool and going for a walk. We were going to be shuttled to and from our appointment destinations, so there was no need to rent a car. Our chosen hotel was located on the edge of an industrial park and around two miles from the local shopping and eating establishments. Unfortunately, the shuttle services, which move to the downtown area and Mayo, do not run on Sundays, so our

111

only option became walking. The weather was beautiful so walking to the local store for a couple of forgotten supplies was great. After shopping and having stopped at a local eatery for lunch, we made it back to the hotel, clocking 4.4 miles on the Fitbit. I am sure the walk did us good, however I was reminded the next morning that I had a knee problem. I had strained it earlier that year and walking for extended times seems to flare it up again. Oh well, this too will serve as a distraction.

The day of our first appointment for a blood draw arrived. We decided to go to Mayo early and take the patient tour. This would familiarize us with the shuttle service, building layouts, and timelines for moving about. Off we went on the shuttle for a 25-minute ride. As you approach the Mayo campus, you realize the enormity of this site. It encompasses the majority of the downtown district, and we later learned it has 35,000 employees at this campus alone.

Walking in the front door, you quickly realize that you are their focus, through the welcoming atmosphere and ever helpful volunteers and staff. We attended the new patient orientation and tour, which was focused on the art, architecture, and history of the Mayo Clinic. We were hoping it would have had more of a medical focus but were pleasantly surprised to learn of the history and commitment of the organization.

Their motto speaks volumes to their organization. **"The best interest of the patient is the only interest to be considered"** were the words and ideology spoken by Dr. William Mayo. I was certain from the limited contact we had experienced to date, that these are not just words on a wall, but have been ingrained into all employees.

We made our way over to the information library dedicated to cancer. In there, we discovered a plethora of information related to any type of cancer you may be experiencing. The attending staff was helpful in identifying and directing us to the information related to prostate cancer, along with providing listings of additional resources we may want to seek out.

As we browsed the other sections, there were two areas of interest for me. One was a section dedicated to prevention and wellness. The information there was not specific to any form of illness, more to a general set of guidelines one should follow. Picking up several pieces of literature, I was eager to see what I may have been doing right or wrong.

The other section that drew my attention was the area of pancreatic cancer. A dear friend of ours was immersed in this disease at that time and was fighting the battle. His current prognosis was not promising, so I wanted to garner any additional information or resource that could be beneficial. Their section on this subject was limited, however helpful.

On the other side of the hall from this resource center lies a room which is dedicated to clinical trials programs. Entering, I was again greeted by a helpful staff member who directed me through the process of finding my desired topic. Exclaiming that I was interested in pancreatic cancer, she proceeded to share several publications and directed me to their web resource that gives a complete listing of the research being done. As treatments advance for the different types of cancer, more energies and brain power are directed toward finding relief and cure for these debilitating diseases. Pancreatic cancer has always been and continues to be one of the least survivable forms of cancer. Mayo currently has extensive research dedicated toward finding a cure for this and are making tremendous advancements. I couldn't wait to share this with our friend.

Realizing that by the time we took the shuttle back to the hotel, it would be time to ride it back to the clinic, we simply nestled in for our upcoming blood work appointment. We were sitting in the lobby watching the ebb and flow of humanity pass through its doors—people whose common bond was seeking answers to the problems they are facing. After a few minutes, we had this shocking revelation that we should go to our assigned department where the blood was going to be drawn and wait there. After all, maybe they would take us early. Amazingly, but not surprising, they checked us in, and I had the blood work drawn within five minutes.

Back to the hotel, we settled in for the evening. Marilyn, while browsing the internet, checked in to the patient portal and discovered the test results were already posted. PSA 4.9—up 2 points from the previous test around 20 days ago. This indicated that it was aggressively climbing and was a source of concern. They measure the aggressiveness of recurrent prostate cancer using a doubling scale. It is the amount of time that it takes for your rising PSA to double. Typically, aggressive forms are doubling in 3-5 months. Mine was doubling in days, 30 to be exact. Drifting off to sleep, we both realized it would be a restless night, again.

The following morning, we arose early as neither of us could sleep. Not so much from the concern over the possible outcome, but again waking up to an unknown journey. We were both focused on having faith—more importantly, having a *knowing* faith—that this was just another journey we had to walk out. The unknown was identifying the path to be taken and we were beginning that walk.

We were both fortunate that we had the ability to take our jobs with us. By simply having a computer and a connection to the internet, we could transform any room or space into an office. So, up in the morning and off to work we went, albeit a couple of steps to the desk and logging on, and we were there. This allowed us to stay busy, productive, and it also served as a diversion. After working for a while, showering, and heading down to breakfast, we were again ready for the adventure. Interestingly, the vast majority of the people at this hotel were somehow connected to Mayo. Most were patients, a few were visitors, and a few had business dealings with the organization.

While sitting at the pool, having breakfast, or on the shuttle, you will meet people who have a story to tell. Some without regard to who is listening, others who are keeping it inside, and then there are those who will share theirs and express interest in yours. We met all types on this journey and feel blessed in both the receiver and the giver roll. Sometimes a simple "I'll be thinking of you" is all that is required to enable a person to continue on. We have been blessed during these interactions, along with the words of encouragement shared through social media. It is easy to forget that you do not have to be walking this out alone. I am not talking about excluding God, yet sometimes we do,

115

but more about others who genuinely care. I know we care for them, and I should never get to a place where I think my gifts of compassion, caring, and concern are greater than anyone else's. Therefore, their words of encouragement were well received and appreciated.

To the clinic we went. Arriving just 45 minutes before our scheduled appointment, we were getting better at this timing thing. We moved quickly to our designated floor where we checked in. The staff again was exemplary, showing concern for our needs and informing us that the doctor was running a little behind, as usual, but would be with us as soon as possible. For some, this would be irritating, after all my time is just as important as his. To us, it is comforting, knowing that there is a doctor who is willing to invest himself in a patient, allowing the time required for the obvious questions that must arise. We are all on a journey we never expected and to finally be in a place where answers can and will be delivered is, in itself, comforting.

The initial meeting was a bit unusual. Dr. Kwon came into the room around the time his Physician's Assistant (PA), a colleague, came in also. They introduced themselves and he casually sat on the footstool of the examination bench, crossing his legs, and getting comfortable. After a brief introduction process, he questioned why we were having this appointment since the C-11 PET scan had not been performed. His logic was sound, as there is a protocol that they follow, however we had managed to come in the backdoor.

We explained that we were there to get all the scans and tests, which were scheduled, but that the insurance company had denied the pre-certification request, pending a peer-to-peer review between he and their doctor. In order for that process to happen, we would need to have been seen by him. So, to facilitate that, we had scheduled an appointment kind of in the wrong order. He fully understood, exchanged pleasantries, and passed us over to the PA for the continuation of the appointment. Even in this short interaction, we could tell he was a caring and knowledgeable person.

The PA was very helpful and understanding of our situation. We asked questions about getting our other scheduled tests moved up. She reviewed the documentation we had provided and discussed options for the pre-certification process, along with who can and should do what. To our amazement, she was fairly matter-of-fact about getting the C-11 scan approved. Typically, if a carrier has declined the procedure, it is a very difficult journey to get that decision reversed. They have had several people accomplish this, but only after hounding them into submission. To this, we acknowledged that we were up to the task and we would do whatever was needed to get it passed. The remaining portion of the appointment was centered around scheduling, fact finding, and strategies in dealing with the insurance carrier. They had scheduled the peer-to-peer for the following day and after that meeting, we would be prepared to file an appeal and begin pushing. Before we left, she had managed to move the MRI up to the following evening.

Retiring again to our hotel, we then proceeded to dive into more research. One of the documents Marilyn had discovered was the guidance document used by our insurance company in making their decision and referenced when denying the requested treatment. This document was available online and we downloaded it for our records. We also reached out to our insurance agent/advocate and explained the issue along with what we felt were going to be challenges in getting the approval. She agreed that it would most likely be an uphill battle and that we should begin preparing our case and forwarding these documents to her in preparation. We were also to reach out to Mayo for a document that stated that Medicare had approved this type of test and deemed it medically necessary. This she believed would go a long way toward supporting our case. Mayo, as advanced of an organization as they are, does not pass documents electronically. I suspect it has to do with security concerns, both for the patient and their organization. However, it required we go there in person to pick up the document. Another shuttle ride and another opportunity to interact with people on their journey.

After returning, I reviewed the guidance document and identified all of the references to C-11 and PET scans. To our amazement, it became apparent there were conflicting statements spread throughout the text. In some cases, it stated it was not necessary and in others it was. We used the document to make our case. We created a guidance document of our own and routed it to both the Mayo PA, who was going to make the peer-to-peer call, and to our insurance advocate, along with supporting information.

As the afternoon unfolded, we sporadically checked the Mayo Clinic portal app and, as we were getting ready to leave the hotel for the scheduled MRI, a simple note was posted stating, "Talked with insurance doctor, test approved, and we are attempting to reschedule quickly!" After a few seconds of digesting these words, we both felt such a sense of relief that the tears welled up. I am not sure which was more important, the idea that our testing was approved, moving us closer to answers, or the sense of relief knowing a battle will not need to be fought. Either way, we were extremely relieved as we boarded the bus.

My MRI was scheduled for late in the day. We did not realize how late until we arrived in the bustling facility to see a thinning crowd. The waiting room had only a few people sitting and waiting. After careful examination, we realized they were waiting for patients to return from their scan and not patients waiting to be processed. "Dave Fuller" was called over the intercom shortly after we checked in, and off we went. First stop, the medical nurse who prepped and inserted the IV line after going over the checklist of "NOTS." No metal, implants, surgical staples, or anything that could be inadvertently ripped out of your body by the extreme magnetic fields of the scanner. Next, to a waiting room where Marilyn and I chatted about how blessed we were and how satisfied we felt with the decision to come to Mayo.

Soon, another technician came in and had me go into a dressing room where I got rid of all clothing and donned the proverbial gown and robe. Back to the waiting room and a lesson on the idiosyncrasies of wearing a skirt from Marilyn. Who knew that it was not cool to cross your legs while wearing a skirt or dress? Thankfully, we were the only ones in the waiting room. Soon the imaging technician came in and escorted me into the MRI room. Reviewing the "NOTS" list again, she briefly described

119

the process. Lay on your side on this table, have a probe shoved up your butt, spin to your back, insert earplugs, have the preliminary scan, adjust as instructed, and then lie still for an hour. Nodding that I understood, we embarked on this journey. Thank goodness she was a kind and cute technician, because if she had been stern and burly, during that part where she shoved the probe in would have been unbearably embarrassing if I would have started crying. Oh, by the way, after it is inserted, there is a balloon that gets inflated to hold it in place. Ouch!

Lying on my back, I was moved into the huge tube, and the scans began. MRI scans are a crazy symphony of whirring, clicking, and bumping. After an initial scan, in she came, removed me from the tube and announced, "I need to reposition the probe and place it next to the prostate." OH BOY, deflate, twist, inflate, and back in the tube. Sounds easy on paper, but it's a little more harsh and involved in person.

Again, the noises, along with a brief stop where she placed additional ear protection on my head. Lying on a table motionless is a difficult task. Having to do it for an hour inside a featureless tube with the feeling you need to have a bowel movement takes an immense amount of will power. The thing I focused on is how important it is to get quality imaging to determine the next course of action. One hour in the grand scheme of things is a small moment in time. I can get through this. After the scans were over, it was out of the tube, probe removed, cleaned up, and dressed. Leaving the facility, it became very real how late this appointment was. We were literally the last non-staff out of the building. The waiting rooms were empty. The lobby only had an occasional cleaning person going about their assigned task. The rotary doors were shut down and the pass door latches had been released. Once you walked out, you were out for the night.

Later that evening, we checked the portal and found the C-11 scan had been moved to the upcoming Friday. Somehow, they had managed to slot us into an opening, which would allow us to have all of our appointments, tests, and scans completed in a week. Understanding that it normally would take weeks to get scheduled into routine scans, we were again amazed at how in tune with a patient's needs this organization is. We are truly blessed in our lives and more importantly thankful for those blessings.

There was a dear friend who was traveling for work in the Twin Cities. He offered to drive to Rochester, around two hours, to meet us for dinner. After enjoying a great meal and good conversation, we were able to FaceTime with his wife, our God Daughter, and their kids before he had to leave. Even when you are traveling, God has a way of keeping the important things and people in your life, if you are open.

The next morning was pretty much free. This was good, as we both had work to get done. Logging into the hotel WIFI, we were able get caught up with the critical needs of work. Realizing we could actually work for a while, we moved our "offices" over to the Mayo building where there is a work area that sort of resembles a desk. This placed us in the building where the next appointment to see Dr. Kwon would take place in the afternoon. With the time change, we somehow got confused and went to the waiting room early. After checking in and realizing we would be there for a while, we were pleasantly surprised when they called my name after waiting only a few minutes.

Meeting with the team, we reviewed the results of the MRI and discovered it returned inconclusive results. Nothing unusual showed up with the prostate, although there was a small bony island on my right hip. The initial assessment indicated that it did not appear to be malignant; however, it was slightly larger than the scan done in 2014. Something worth looking at on the C-11 scan for sure. Bottom line, it gave more credence to our decision to use the C-11 scan.

Determining that the scan would be tomorrow, Friday, and that the results would not be available until Monday morning, we were excited to plan our exit from the Mayo area for a while. We decided it would be appropriate to rent a car and go back to Indiana. There we could be with family, get back to work, and wait for the call with the results of the scan. Our need to meet face-to-face with the team was not required at this time. They were going to review the data, determine the next possible courses of action, and call us for consultation. If there was a need to return to Mayo, we would be able to schedule the needed appointments and make the trip back. For now, after tomorrow's scan, we needed to step back for a while.

The next morning, we began our typical day with breakfast and work. We checked out of the hotel late morning and headed over to Mayo to set up our "offices." They offer a bag check service where we could drop our luggage, which we did. We identified where our appointment was and proceeded to the waiting room. After making sure we knew the procedure and the timing, we made our way to the library in this part of the Mayo complex, located on the subway level, where we could set up our computers to get some work done. We were pleasantly surprised to again find work stations that well suited our needs. There, we again accomplished the demands for the day before we headed up to the waiting room and checked in.

The C-11 scan I was scheduled for is a unique type of scan, not in terms of the imaging equipment, but rather in the IV injection required. As explained earlier, it is an isotope created in a cyclotron, located on site. This is then attached to the Choline molecule which is then injected into your body. The tracer only has a 20-minute half-life, so it quickly loses its effectiveness. To perform the test then, you are required to be in the scanner, waiting for the liquid to be delivered. When they called my name, I was escorted to the IV insertion room, where a nurse again poked a needle in my arm. I had not been drinking much that morning, so finding a vein seemed more difficult this time. After searching both arms, he chose a desired spot and began poking toward the vein. Missing it, he pulled the needle part way out and attempted a different angle. After repeating this process, I'm guessing, 15 times, he exclaimed, "If this hurts, let me know."

My response was, "Shouldn't you have told me this before you started using me as a pin cushion?"

He laughed and said, "Oh yeah, sorry."

After abandoning this site completely and wrapping the wound, he moved to another site and started the process over. Still not able to successfully hit a vein, he declared he would get another more experienced nurse to complete the process. I felt somewhat relieved when the next nurse came in and after only two quick pokes, had the IV in place.

They announced that the imaging technician would be in soon and, as they were finishing the sentence, she was walking in. Off we went to the scanner where she announced the C-11 was going to be in the room at 2 pm. We had little time to get all set up in the scanner. It felt unusual that I was not required to change clothes. I simply needed to assure them there was no metal in my pockets or elsewhere, which would distort the scan. That was easy, just remove my belt and lay on the table. Passing me through the scanner to determine that all cushions and limbs would not interfere, I was repositioned at the starting point where I waited for the magic fluid to arrive.

A three-minute wait was all that was required. Giving me a few final instructions as she injected the fluid, she removed the IV from my arm, exited the room, and the scan began. This scan was only 25 minutes scan, so it was quickly over. Rising from the table, I was directed to the exit. Out to the waiting room, Marilyn and I felt a sense of relief, knowing we were leaving the area and going back to Indiana for some R and R.

We decided that our preferred method of getting to the airport, where the car rental company was located, would be Uber. We had never used this service before and found the entire process easy to navigate. Use the app on your phone, hail a ride, post a payment, and get in the vehicle when it arrives. The ride was quick and comfortable, driven by a young gentleman who was a musician and just liked to drive. Arriving at the airport, we got our rental car and left. The trip, of eight-plus hours, forced us to decide if we were going to stop on the way or just drive straight through. We opted to drive through and arrived at our son's house at 1:00 am.

Saying brief greetings, we slipped into our room and welcomed the inviting pillows to our heads as we drifted off to sleep. We both slept well, albeit short, knowing that this pause in the process would again be broken come Monday when the expected "results" call would come in, hopefully beginning our charting of the new path toward a new action phase. We were both feeling confident in our decision to include Mayo in our journey. But for now, a little peace and a lot of family time was needed.

Being back in Indiana with friends and family was definitely therapeutic. It is always wonderful to see our son and his new girlfriend, and Marilyn was especially happy to reconnect with her sisters. While we thoroughly enjoy our new lives in Florida, the people we left behind all have special places in our hearts. I do not know any better feeling than being with loved ones, especially when there are challenges ahead. The support mechanisms, which were fostered earlier, had become a vital component to coping with the stress of the unknown. Simply getting back to the normality of life allowed us to place the "cancer" topic on hold, giving us a chance to collect our thoughts and reflect. So there we were, enjoying life, and celebrating Mother's Day with our son.

The weekend passed quickly and soon we found ourselves back in the thick of job-hood. Since we were in town, it was appropriate to go into the office where we could experience a real workstation. Knowing that we could be called any minute with the test results, which may change our plans at any moment, was uncomfortable. They had committed to call us on Monday and if that did not happen, we were to call them on Tuesday.

So here we were in the waiting game again, exactly where unlimited stress can materialize.. My best methodology for coping with this is to preoccupy myself with routine tasks. This is in no way a denial of the situation, but rather a healthy way to allow the time to pass productively. I literally take it out of my mind and table it for a while. Once sufficient time has passed, I will reach out and pick it up, verify the status, and react to whatever is presented. If nothing is to be done or learned, I place it back on the table and move on.

During one of those moments, I logged onto the patient portal and discovered that the images of the test, along with the technician's assessment, was posted. Knowing that we are not trained medical professionals and that we would leave the final interpretation to the doctor, we anxiously opened the report.

Bottom line, four areas of concern had shown up as possible malignancies, two with high probability and two that were suspicious. The news was actually welcoming. To have gone through all of the testing and come out with all inconclusive results would have been far worse than finding something. That option would only mean waiting until it had grown sufficiently to be detected and again being mired in that horrible waiting game. At least with these results, our conclusion, albeit amateuristic, was that we would be able to focus curative energies toward a specific set of targets. Now the anxiousness stepped up a few notches.

Monday came and went without a call. Tuesday would be the day. "Hurry up and call." At work, we busied ourselves with the tasks at hand. Occasionally, I would realize that time had passed without a call and would wonder what the holdup was. Realizing that there was ample time to get the answers we were anticipating, I would return my focus to work. Then Marilyn would call me to ask if I had heard anything yet. Responding that I had not, I could hear the disappointment in her voice as she muttered, "Let me know as soon as you do!" Acknowledging that I would, we each drifted back into our work. Soon it was around noon and still no answer.

The call to Mayo went in and I was informed that the doctor had been notified that the results were posted and would contact us when he had a chance to review them. He had not been "in clinic" the previous day which was contrary to what he had expected and, therefore, was running behind. Also, he was leaving for a conference on Wednesday and would need to get to us by the end of the day or wait until Monday when he returned. This call to them happened four more times before we were informed that he may make the call after hours and to be patient.

The day ended with no answer and with our first small disappointment. While I was confident that the information would be conveyed to us all within the timeframes that would allow treatment to be administered, the fact was we were in this waiting land with potential answers so close that it hurt. Somehow, there was an understanding that we would not be able to do anything toward a treatment plan until the following week when he returned, yet we still were on the edge of this precipice and left hanging.

I deal with this type of situation much differently than Marilyn does. She will not rest until the answers are provided and will carry that stress with her. I dismiss the stress by allowing the forces to work while keeping a mindful eye on the situation—again, like laying it down for a while and picking it back up when I feel the time is right. There is nothing wrong with either of these approaches; however, it is wrong to drag the other into my world. I must allow her to process in her way, as she must allow me to process in mine. Therein is where our peace exists, and stress is managed. Tomorrow will be another day and we will continue the pursuit.

Chapter 8

The New Path

Another typical day began with the normal routine of up in the morning, off to work, busy with the day's events, and waiting for the call. This day was a bit unusual because I was needed at a remote building where the service provider was scheduled to install the communications/internet connections. Being at this site meant there was not a direct connect, which would allow me to do work and, therefore, also had no easy way to keep up with potential emails and/or posts from the clinic. After a few hours with no call, I called the clinic again as a gentle reminder, only to be informed that the doctor and nurse were out of the building and not expected to return until Wednesday of the following week. This was exactly a week away, so the realization that we may not have answers until then dimmed my spirit.

Thirty minutes later, I received a call from one of the team members who had been instructed to give me the results of their conversation the previous evening. After brief introductions and pleasantries, it was down to business. "Mr. Fuller, the scan had picked up a few areas of concern. One on the humorous, another in the pelvic area, two others in the tail bone and hip area. We would like to schedule a consult next week where we can address any issues, lay out a treatment regimen, and begin the process toward healing." The rest of the conversation went on to work out the details and get the ball rolling.

Finally, we were getting answers. I am not going to say that these were the desired answers, but they were welcome. To go through these processes and not have definitive targets would have been disappointing. I suppose there would have been a case to understand that God had already facilitated the cure and removed it from my body, but there would have been the doubt that the scan just did not see it yet. Thank God we had a decisive answer that now moved us closer to the cure. I called Marilyn and her expression of relief brightened my spirit. Now all we needed to do was to go through the motions and get ourselves to Mayo in a week. Our job now was to stay positive and focused on our destination.

There had been a brief mention that the treatment may include chemotherapy along with other options. Chemo and its side effects now became a topic of investigation. I was not versed in its effects or methodologies. We scheduled an appointment with the urologist at Mayo the following week for first thing in the morning. The waiting room was empty, not a soul to be seen. The registration desk which was typically staffed by two to three attendants was eerily vacant. Everything had been cleaned and picked up the night before by the custodial staff, and we almost felt guilty even wanting to sit down and wait for fear we would move something out of its place or ruffle a seat. Realizing we were around twenty minutes early, we made ourselves comfortable to wait for the staff to appear and check us in.

After a brief, maybe five minute, wait, the exam room doors opened and Dr. Kwon strolled out and paged "Mr. Fuller!" The irony of that was humorous as we looked around to a completely empty room. Standing and working our way toward him, we exchanged greetings and moved to his office for our appointment. Somehow, this small but genuine gesture of him coming in early and personally greeting us at the door, enhanced the opinion and respect we were developing for this man, again solidifying our decision to come to this place.

Sitting in his office, he reviewed my chart, reading aloud, re-familiarizing himself with the images as he began discussing the findings. One primary lesion located inside the top of the left arm bone, one small undetermined spot on the tail bone and a few other suspicious areas to be determined were found. He exclaimed that it was definitely unusual to find prostate cancer metastasized in an arm bone, however, it was not unheard of and, more importantly, it was good news.

Going on, he explained that it is always much better to find a large growth located in a fairly confined area, as the treatment becomes much more targeted. With a little smile on his face, he simply stated, "We just need to zap that, and I suspect your PSA will diminish greatly or even go to zero. While we are at it, we should consult with the radiation oncologist and see if he would also target the spot on the tail bone as an added insurance policy. The remaining suspicious spots would then be placed on a watch list and targeted as needed. This process would be

133

appropriate even if a wider distribution of cancer cells is detected at a later date, as any systemic type treatment would have greater success if the large known pockets are eradicated first." His recommendation was to refer us to Dr. Park, a radiation oncologist on staff at Mayo, who he credits as being one of the best in the world in his field. Knowing the caliber of the staff here, I believe he probably is. And having peers attest to each other's abilities again provides more assurance.

After a brief discussion, we informed him that we had just recently lost our good friend to pancreatic cancer and that we were leaving, following this meeting, to go back to Indiana for his funeral. We sensed a little disappointment as he was preparing to kick start the process to get this nipped in the bud right away. Dictating instructions to his staff to set up an MRI of the shoulder, forward the images and findings to the radiation oncologist for review and consult, and set up appointments for follow-up meetings, he finally took us to the post-appointment staff member, who had just gotten situated for the day, to finalize the details. We thanked him for coming in early and parted ways.

We waited for the rest of the clinic to come to life to confirm our next steps. The staff member who was working with us came to the lobby and let us know it was going to take some time to get everything set, as the precursory swipe at it hit an obstacle with the insurance company. They denied the use of an MRI on the shoulder to diagnose prostate cancer and prepare it for treatment. Now, when it is stated that way, you need to step back and laugh along with them. This does testify to the unusualness of this type of cancer reappearing in these areas.

What this meant to us was more battles with the insurance company. It seemed the learned, highly trained puppets who work for the insurance company that controls the money, knew with much greater certainty what procedures or treatments should be applied, better than the masters themselves. None-the-less, we were handcuffed by the process and would continue to play the game. We left for the nine-hour drive home, occasionally reaching out to those who were playing along with us, to confirm all was moving forward. At the conclusion of the day, the one positive thing we could hang our hat on was there would be another peer-to-peer call tomorrow which should clear the way forward.

It never ceases to amaze me how complexity creeps into any situation whenever people are involved. What seems like a simple process, make a call, get an approval, somehow transforms itself into not just another event, but rather a journey of its own. The phone call never materialized because the pre-certification could only be approved inside a certain window prior to the scheduled appointment. The appointment could not be scheduled because the pre-certification had not been approved.

The only outcome then was to schedule the appointments into the nearest available opening, which suited all parties if urgency was not considered. This placed the appointment out thirty-five days. AAAAGGGGHHH! With the sense of urgency that had been conveyed to us through our conversations with Dr. Kwon, this became another point of anxiety. The only thing we could do was to step into the seemingly simple process and take back control.

After we made phone calls to the pre-certification department, the urology department, the insurance agent, then the pre-cert department again, then urology, the pre-cert, urology, insurance, and finally the urology department again, we managed to put the pieces of the puzzle together and get the peer-to-peer call made. This achieved the pre-certification approval, which lead to the scheduling of the appointments all within the following week. Five appointments all scheduled on the same day, including the radiation simulation required to determine the exact treatment methodology and setup. With this complete, the next step would be a special kind of targeted radiation called Stereotactic Body Radiation Therapy (SBRT). We were confident that those appointments would be following while we were at the clinic.

Not assuming anything, we remained in the center of the process. Traveling to Mayo always involved overnight stays. This required booking a hotel and without a firm, or anticipated schedule, we were kind of shooting in the dark. So, the next calls were to the clinic in an attempt to define the length of stay to assist in making those reservations. We understood the challenge of trying to pin this down as the radiation oncologist had not even seen our charts, so he would not be able to make a definitive or even estimated call. However, we made the calls and attempted to define it based on "guestimates" from past cases. Who knows, we may get it right. Until then, we relaxed, prayed, meditated, and continued our journey.

From Indiana/Michigan to Rochester, Minnesota on the GPS it says you are in for a six hour and forty-seven minute trip. If you could ever drive the speed limit, without any delays or breaks for gas or food, I believe the timeline would be correct. I, like anyone else who may be reading this, do not live inside one of those boxes. We happen to live in the real world where the unexpected is expected. With our upcoming schedule of doctor's appointments looming, we decided that it would be wise to get an early jump on the trip. Leaving the morning of the day before, we managed to squeeze the six hour forty-seven minute trip into eight hours and fifteen minutes. Having traveled this route several times before, we were glad to get there safely and to have time to check into the hotel for a bit of rest before the next morning's early start.

There are many, and I do mean many, hotels in and around Rochester. While there are other businesses and industries located here, Mayo is by far the primary purpose for travelers to be in Rochester. This requires a litany of lodges which can flex and contract as the demand for housing breathes. Unlike most locations which have rates which reflect demand, this area operates backwards from your typical hotels. At most hotels, during the week you will find the cheapest rates and on the weekends, the more expensive ones. This law of supply and demand works because people are traveling to areas where they will be on vacations.

Rochester, however, is a destination, not for pleasure but rather for life. People are coming here to identify and treat issues which would get in the way of vacation traveling. I mention this because I have found it interesting how the laws of free market and capitalism work in all aspects of our lives. The laws of supply and demand find a way to balance themselves if left to their own forces

137

without intervention. Because of the diversity of available establishments, the costs in Rochester remain affordable.

Organizations whose missions are to support the afflicted, are prevalent in the area and provide support and options for those who cannot afford the stays. As we have experienced, the appointments breed appointments when you are seeking answers. One night can quickly turn into five and beyond. The average individual will find themselves racking up a considerable amount of costs, simply waiting around for their next appointment.

These organizations have become the source of hope for many. They provide housing to many through donations of others, allowing people, who would simply have to leave the area, to stay and seek life. Sometimes we have a tendency to take these organizations for granted and believe that they somehow just exist. They do not and will not exist without the generosity of others who have chosen to support them and their causes. The small act of helping someone find a restful night's sleep, allows a searching soul time to find their answers. To those who have donated and to those who will, a huge thank you and blessings. To myself, I feel a stronger need to reach out to these organizations and offer support.

Because of the early morning appointment, we were outside the scope of the shuttle systems. We needed to be at the clinic forty minutes before the first shuttle was scheduled to leave the hotel. Setting the alarms for 4:45 am, we were up, around, and waiting for the 5:30 am beginning of breakfast. With a full day of appointments scheduled, we wanted to make sure we had something to eat before our adventures began. Eating quickly, we drove to the clinic, parked, and made our way to the subway level, only to find that the gates were drawn and not scheduled to open until five minutes before our first appointment, the MRI.

After scouting around a little, I found a back door for early hours entry and convinced an employee to let us follow him in. What happened next was a testament to their motto, mentioned before, "The best interest of the patient is the only interest to be considered."

Because we were coming into the building through a foreign route, the building layout was not familiar. We stopped to get our bearings when a gentleman in a white coat approached. "Can I help you?" he asked. After hearing our destination, he proceeded to give us directions. Then, he did something amazing. He simply stood there as if in anticipation of the next question. After a brief uncomfortable lull, we realized that he was not going to leave us if we still had questions. We thanked him for taking the time, and we both parted our separate ways. There, in an early morning meetup, the caring concern that they are known for became apparent.

We then made our way up to the imaging waiting room and managed to check in when the first staff appeared a good ten minutes before the scheduled time. If we have learned anything along this path, it is to be resourceful and not get caught up in the details or obstacles. Years ago, one of our pastors used a statement, "Blessed be the flexible for they won't be bent out of shape" in one of his sermons. This has become a life lesson to us and an understanding that things will not always go as planned. We must simply persevere and move on.

MRI, doctor appointment/initial meeting with radiation oncologist, best in his field, Dr. Park, then radiation simulation, interview assessment, blood work, and finally a meeting with Dr. Kwon, our urologist. Beginning at 6:15 in the morning and ending up at 4:30 in the afternoon, the amount of information to be processed continued to build. IV lines placed, scans done, and then IVs pulled. Body casts made and CT scans done, questionnaires filled out, needles to draw blood inserted, and finally a relaxing (not) time discussing the findings, and a follow-up plan loaded with medical terms. By the end of the day, when we checked our appointment schedule on the patient portal, we had three SBRT radiation treatments scheduled for the following week.

Now, the decision had to be made on whether we travel back to Indiana or stay in Rochester? Traveling eight-plus hours for the weekend was attractive, as we would be back close with some friends and family; however, we would then need to turn around and drive back. Staying in the hotel over the weekend seemed monotonous and another source of money drain. Another option crept into our thoughts, which was to drive north to visit a friend who was recovering from a fall. This seemed like the preferred choice, and we made plans to make the trip.

Our friend had recently gone through a divorce and, during the moving process, he had fallen down a flight of stairs. Arriving at the bottom, he had eight broken ribs and a punctured lung. Being there alone, he managed to sit himself upright but was unable to move any further. He could only wait and hope he would be found. Over an hour later, a concerned neighbor located him and called

911 to summon help. Barely clinging to life, he was airlifted to Duluth, Minnesota where they managed to keep him alive. After recovering for a few weeks, he was released to a regional rehab facility for his recuperation. This nursing home/rehab facility was not good for him. Ultimately, he ended back in the local hospital with pneumonia, presumably from the healing punctured lung. This was a great opportunity for us to deflect our attention from our plight and go to see him, while enjoying the summertime scenery of upper Wisconsin. Little did we know, this would also turn into a journey itself.

We chose to stay off the interstate system and wandered along the trip by taking two lane state highways, which passed through several cute little towns. We really did not have a deadline other than needing to be back at Mayo on Monday morning for my first treatment. The rolling countryside of the state is extremely beautiful. If you can picture the mid-growth crops swaying gently in a breeze, wandering up and over rolling hills. In the distance a farmstead, impeccably cared for, nestled in a quiet valley with a few trees providing shade from the sun, radiating in the clear blue sky. Next to the home, sat the barn and silos, waiting patiently for the autumn crops to be delivered for their safe keeping. As we peered in the distance, this scene repeated itself over and over until the farm disappeared behind us into the horizon. Each bend in the road opened this repeating picture and made the trip of four hours seem to pass effortlessly.

As we got closer to our destination, we received a call from his daughter who informed us that he had been getting progressively worse and that an ambulance was going to transport him back to Duluth for care more appropriate to his needs. Just our luck, we thought, to drive the morning only to see him loaded into an ambulance for transport far away. Now we would need to decide if we stay and sightsee or turn around and go back. But once we got to the hospital, we had mixed emotions when we found out he was being held pending the return of the transport from a prior emergency run to the same hospital in Duluth. The trip there and back would take them around five hours, which allowed us visitation time, but delayed his much needed treatment. However, it was nice to spend that time with him and his daughter and her family.

Realizing that his condition was serious, we decided to make the trek to Duluth so we could be there when he was admitted. His daughter was traveling there that evening to be with him, and we wanted to be there to support them both. We arrived at the hospital around thirty minutes before the transport got there. Once he was in the room, the doctors began the methodical process of determining his status and formulating a plan toward healing. Being the closest thing to family at that time, they were asking us questions about his condition. Our assistance was extremely limited, and we were careful not to attempt to speak of things we didn't know, but we were able to fill in a few blanks until his daughter arrived.

After xrays and tests, the doctors determined he had excess fluid built up around his lungs, along with an infection in that fluid. They inserted a drain tube while we were there and placed him on antibiotics. We all felt confident he was now getting good care.

We had trouble getting a hotel room for the evening, because there was an air show in town, and all rooms were either booked and/or expensive. We finally managed to find an affordable room around thirty miles outside of town. Checking in for the evening, we were glad for a semi-comfortable bed and the anticipation of a good night's sleep.

The following morning, we got up and moseyed back into town to the hospital to find him resting much more comfortably. He was far from being out of the woods but was most definitely on a much better path. After visiting awhile, we said our goodbyes and well wishes and left the hospital to head home, or at least back to Mayo, our temporary home.

Seizing on this unexpected opportunity to visit a beach, we managed to make our way to the shoreline of Lake Superior. Duluth sits on the very western most tip of this Great Lake and, because of that, is somewhat unique. Years ago, we began the tradition of collecting sand from significant destination beaches along our travels. We would purchase a shot glass from the local area, place the sand and a unique shell or stone from that beach in it and keep it as a memento of our travels. Gathering some sand and a couple of the flattened stones from the beach, we found a tourist-type shop that had a shot glass worthy of holding our treasure. This would be a welcome contribution to our collection and a reminder of our small, yet significant, side trip to support a friend in need. Heading back on the four-hour trip to Mayo felt good, knowing that we were moving toward my treatment at last.

The American Cancer Society (ACS) has long been an organization that has created programs to support cancer victims and their families. These include their supportive, caring, gentle-hearted volunteers, their financial support for research, their informational literature, and their housing programs for those who are undergoing treatment. The latter of these manifests itself in support housing located near the treatment facilities. These places provide a safe environment where patients and their families can rest and recover from the treatment's side effects.

Needing to stay close to the treatment facilities can and does become a drain financially on many, including us. The ACS provides this housing free of charge, through the generous donations of others, through volunteer staff, and through resident contributions. These support homes are typically in high demand due to the number of patients who are typically seeking treatment and has risen greatly over the last several decades. To manage the overflow, the ACS has reached out to local hotels who have graciously offered to provide significantly discounted rates for those who are waiting for lodging in one of the support homes. Because of our treatment cycles, we qualified for the lodging and, therefore, the discounted rates. We had contacted one of the local hotels and booked our rooms for a 50% saving over the published room rates. Knowing we would be there for several days and that there was a potential for side effects, we upgraded slightly to a King Suite. The primary reason for this was the inclusion of a couch where we could rest comfortably. Arriving back in Rochester, we checked in and got settled for the evening in anticipation of the next morning's scheduled treatment.

The next morning, we were up, dressed, went downstairs for breakfast, and then waited for the shuttle bus to ferry us to the clinic. The shuttle service is managed like clockwork. At exactly 7:25 am, its scheduled time, the shuttle pulled up in front of the hotel. We, along with several others, piled into the bus. Our appointment this time was not in the clinic but rather in an adjoining hospital. There is a walking subway system which interconnects these facilities; however, we chose to walk outside along the sidewalks. The weather was beautiful and getting a chance to enjoy the outdoors is always welcome.

Arriving at the hospital, we checked in at the appropriate desk. Glancing around, we realized that this is a place of hope. Fellow patients were checking in, waiting patiently, sharing stories, and heading back for treatments. All of them have one thing on their mind. **Healing!** When their radiation treatments are complete, there will be a part of them, albeit an unwelcome part, destroyed forever. What is the compelling reason for subjecting ourselves to the killing rays? To choose life—to extend our lives to accomplish more of what God has placed us here for.

The idea is that living is a choice. I have always known this, and it has been my attitude throughout my life. Sometimes, though, it becomes easy to get consumed in the process and not enjoy the journey. To see others walking this out through their own personal challenges is uplifting. I have acquaintances who would sit in these waiting rooms and see the disease and suffering. This would become their object of focus. Soon they would be consumed with negativity to the point of depression. To accept this as reality is defeating and clouds the possibility of joy. Instead, I choose to see hope and the promise of one more day.

The pager vibrates to life and calls you to the appointment desk. There you are directed down the hall toward a waiting assistant. The attendant then directs you to the dressing rooms where the appropriate attire, PJ style pants and a gown are waiting for you. Donning these and locking the room behind you, you wait in the hall corridor for the technician to lead you to the treatment room. Without much wait, you are escorted to the designated room where a large radiation device and a team of technicians are waiting for your arrival. The previously formed mold is laid out on the table and the technicians help you onto it, place the plastic sheeting over you, tuck it in, and turn on the vacuum. The suction quickly draws you down and seals you onto the table. The feeling reminds me of what it would be like to be vacuum sealed.

Adjusting the table to a beginning point, they smiled and reassured me that they are with me all the way and exited the room. Slowly the machine came to life, adjusting, turning, arms extending and retracting, whirring, and bumping until it all quieted down. The machine began its precise rotation around the assigned path, delivering the curative dose of radiation. Two minutes tops was all the time required to kill the cancer in my arm. Amazingly, because of the accurate location of the cancer imaging, it only required one treatment.

Soon, the staff came in and repositioned me for the treatment of the sacral area. The whole process was repeated and when this was finished, they came in and released the vacuum. During the actual treatment time, you are aware that you have been immobilized; however, it is not until they release the seal that you realize how tightly you were held. Simple things like wiggling your toes bring a little glimmer of a smile to your face. They help you out of your cocoon and lead you back to the dressing room. There, you change back into your clothes, discard the fashionable treatment attire, and head out to the waiting room. This entire process took only forty-five minutes. The hours, days. and weeks of analytics, appointments, tests, and preparations were over, at least for my arm, in forty-five minutes. I am not saying that I was disappointed that it did not take longer, but it did seem a bit anticlimactic. For now, I was free to enjoy my day and simply make my way back to the "waiting" room.

After meeting back up with Marilyn, we grabbed a snack from the volunteers who staff a small coffee dispensary to serve the patients. There is an extraordinarily strong presence in Mayo of volunteers who have dedicated a portion of their lives toward providing comfort for those who are suffering. Most are elderly and have been affected by some sort of illness or disease in either themselves or their loved one's lives. Knowing that the professionals at the clinic have the technical portion of an individual's treatment covered, they take on the challenge of providing support and direction to those in need. Their presence is everywhere in the facility and always welcome. Simply having people in the building with you, voluntarily, is again comforting. Whether you are there with someone or by yourself, you are never alone.

Leaving the clinic, we boarded the shuttle bus to return to our temporary residence at the hotel. The remainder of our day was free and with the opportunity to rest, we settled in with our computers to do some much-needed catchup with work.

The next day was a repeat of the first day with a slight variation. They had scheduled an appointment with the radiation oncologist to pass along concerns and information. He reviewed the treatment plan with us, covered potential side effects, defined our follow-up process, and discussed what the team considered their major concerns. The potential side effects for this type of treatment are fatigue, early pain at the treatment site (which diminishes quickly), hair loss (mild), and the possibility of adjacent damage to surrounding tissue. The latter being mentioned only as a disclaimer. The special targeted SBRT radiation is extremely accurate and under the direction of competent doctors, physicists, and technicians, the risks are minimal. Feeling confident in both the process and its players, we left feeling reassured and confident also in the outcome. After the meeting, it was back to the hotel and work.

The morning of the final day, when we woke up, was somehow a little more joyous. We were in the middle of the treatment process, like the days before, but this day was a day we were checking out of the hotel and heading back to Indiana. Knowing that Mayo will continue to be a part of our lives for the near future, we were excited to get back to friends, family, and work. With a treatment time of 1:15 pm and a nine-hour drive ahead of us, we vacillated between driving straight through or stopping along the way. Ultimately, we decided to simply drive until we were tired and stop if needed. I am sure it was the adrenalin that kept us going, but we arrived at our son's house at 11:30

that evening. Happy to finally be in a place where we could simply focus on life and living, we settled in for the night and a welcomed rest.

Chapter 9

The Unexpected

So many well wishes, so many friends, and so many stories. A common theme interlaced throughout this story, as you may have found, is the agony of waiting. I can't emphasize enough that waiting is only one component of the journey and the feeling of helplessness which can go along with it is indicative of your focus. As I have learned on this path, I will move in the direction that my thoughts and mind face. If I get consumed in the need to have answers and patiently wait for them, I may simply stop living and enjoying the life I have. The return from immersing yourself into the search for answers and cures is, therefore, welcome and needed to maintain a sense of balance and to bring life to the hope for a cure. For this understanding, I trust that I will never allow myself to drift into a state of pity or feeling as though I have been cheated by this journey. In fact, it is because of the challenges, that I have been able to enhance these last trips around the sun.

As we began the reinsertion into normality, there were countless opportunities to interact with the afflicted. Each and every one of us has a story and challenges which we face. Having been exposed to affliction myself has opened up a level of understanding and compassion that I had not known previously. God has empowered my gifts of compassion and empathy, along with the gift of helps and discernment so much more in these past few years than ever before. As we meet and reconnect with friends, family, and strangers, I see a person a little differently than before. In converse, they see me differently also. The familiar conversations of the past now take on an unfamiliar element. Those who have heard of our journey approach us with heartfelt concern that I am on the road to recovery. This is sometimes accompanied with a new attitude which has an overtone of pity, albeit not intentional.

A simple, "How are you doing?" can come across in many forms. The difference is in the inflection of their voice or even their mannerisms. The question posed as a genuine concern, simply showing interest, or wanting to gain information, tells me that they are concerned, and is very comforting. The same question presented in a different tone is received as "I am feeling sorry for you." One is presented in an effort to pull you up and the other has the feeling of them pulling you down. I know this is not the intention, but it has served as a reminder to me that my heart should preclude my words in every interaction I have. I ask myself, am I being supportive and compassionate or am I feeling sorry for them? Once I can answer that question, I know how my "How are you doing?" will be perceived. This simple question to myself as a gut check keeps me focused on the direction the conversation will take, up or down. For this understanding, I am extremely grateful.

Work enabled us to get back into a routine while we were in Indiana/Michigan. We all have a life rhythm or heartbeat that feels comfortable to us, and, connected to that heartbeat is a routine which provides us peace. To some, this is a slow soothing rhythm, to others it is a more upbeat tempo. I happen to find myself more at home when the beat is quicker than Marilyn's. For me, to settle into that upbeat pulse, rekindles my sense of purpose. The idea that I am somehow contributing to a greater cause sits well with me and feels comfortable. Being able to work at my job gives me that. It helps me feel that I'm contributing and being productive.

My employer has been an amazing source of comfort to me throughout my cancer journey. I often think back on how wonderful it was that he was able to give me work assignments that could fulfill that sense of purpose for me even during all the required travels for the cancer treatments. Therefore, given the opportunity to show him my appreciation for this, by working every day that I can, also feels great. Marilyn has been supportive, yet still gives me a gentle warning that I am working too much.

After several weeks of working and visiting in the north, we decided that it was time for us to return to our home in the south. We had not been back since the journey to Mayo began. Living out of a carry-on bag for going on two months had been interesting. While we managed it, fairly well I might add, we needed to reload. Our intention was to transition into a snow-bird type of lifestyle with a home in Florida and one in Indiana. Finding a home in Indiana became more of a challenge than we had hoped for, but we were persistent.

We arrived back in Florida to a welcoming of friends and family who were full of questions. While we continued to reach out to them during our absence, there is nothing like the hugs and face to face conversations. This sense of closeness solidifies the bonds and brings us closer.

There is an adage that says "Absence makes the heart grow fonder" which has been a part of conversations for most of my life when someone is not near. This comment is usually given when an important person in your life is missing from your presence. It has a feeling of correctness as you do long for that personal connection even more as time passes. If the person you are longing to connect with is no longer with us, the saying transitions to "Time heals all wounds." Somehow this also feels comforting, knowing that life will move on.

However, the challenge we can face lies in that middle ground where the longing to reconnect becomes unbearable, and the wisdom of knowing when to let go for healing is needed. When the bond is permanently broken, we must let go of it and hang on to our faith. But, most importantly, when the bond is repairable, we need to keep up our hope. Wherever we are in that hard middle ground, the true comfort lies in the knowledge that we are not alone. God, family, and friends all become sources of strength—and rejoicing when we finally move out of that place in our lives.

I had to go through loss at a young age. When I was in High school, my brother who was serving in the Navy, developed Leukemia. He was stationed in Pensacola, Florida and I was overseas attending high school in Taiwan. He was four years my senior, but as children we often had adventures together in the woods near our childhood home. We were not extremely close, but that sibling bond had definitely formed. Separated both in time and physicality, I would long for the time we would come together again. His presence in my life did not diminish over time, in fact there were times when I felt closer to him than ever, even with the separation. He ultimately succumbed to the leukemia. At that moment I was overcome emotionally. I knew that my desire to reconnect would never be fulfilled. So much so that I would sit and cry from the heartache. As time marched on and through God's gentle loving hand, I found peace in knowing that his suffering had ended. I was finally able to start to let go. Knowing that our relationship, while not physical, would remain intact through thoughts and faith, I began the journey toward healing, slowly leaving the grief behind.

Losing someone through death is very hard. Losing someone through rejection can be just as painful, but in a different way. There are times when we can become consumed in the desire to repair a broken relationship to the point where our joy begins to drain. Like God, our desire to reconnect is unending and our hearts and arms are always open, however we must continue to live our lives. This is the place where we find balance in learning how to set it aside temporarily to protect our joy. The reality is a relationship is based on two parties coming together. If the other is not ready or unwilling, then our desire to connect does not diminish, but with God's hand in ours, we can only wait until they are ready also. Love demands that we never close a door and learn patience.

The main lesson we can learn from our losses is to focus on enjoying the good, loving, close relationships we do have with friends and family by having in-person, face to face visits with them. That's what we now had the time and privilege to do in Florida. We deeply enjoyed every minute we could spend with loved ones.

After a month of keeping our southern life assembled, we were back in Indiana. There, we continued our search for a new home and finally found one that would work well for us. Immersed in work, we had our offer accepted and took possession of the home on Labor Day weekend. It needed a little work to bring it up to our standards, but we have never shied away from getting our hands dirty. Cleaning, painting, gardening, and stripping wallpaper became our way of life for the first part of September. This was only going to be short lived, as we had a scheduled follow-up appointment at Mayo, two weeks after closing. When that time arrived, we again jumped in the car and made our 450-mile pilgrimage to the clinic. During that drive, we talked about the remodeling and decorating plans for the new home and made the supportive lists to keep us on track.

The routine at Mayo had become all too familiar. Check into the hotel, go to the clinic for blood work and scans, back to the hotel to work, next day to the clinic for the results and then home. This set of scans returned a result we weren't expecting. "We have found a metastasis on your left hip" took us a little by surprise. I had become good at knowing what is going on in my body and, with no indications of trouble, was fairly confident it would be routine. So much for trusting those feelings. Now we had to move on.

Dr. Kwon confirmed that it was regionalized and very treatable. He made a recommendation of treatment that would include Cryoablation (freezing) surgery of the left

Iliac. It is very comforting to have physicians who have walked this path before and have the wisdom to guide you. After discussing the diagnosis, options, and plans, he picked up the phone and called an associate for a referral. While we were sitting there, they determined that we should come right down (4 floors) and see him immediately.

The Mayo organization continues to amaze me. Typically, in the regular medical field, we would see a physician who would make a diagnosis requiring further analysis or treatment. Next, would be the referral process, along with finding a time in their schedule to get an appointment. This would usually take several days at which time the appointment would be made for several weeks downstream. Next, you would visit Doctor #2 who would require additional tests and would schedule them for a few weeks out. After these tests, you would be back at Doctor #2 to review the results. After determination, they would take a couple of days to schedule the treatment and/or pass you on to Doctor #3 for another evaluation. Once all were on the same page, the treatment would be scheduled, and more weeks would pass. Finally, after six to eight weeks, you would get the treatment/surgery required. Not so at Mayo. Within an hour and a half, we were in front of the next doctor discussing the treatment.

Because the two doctors had talked directly, the scheduling staff had no information on our appointment. We arrived at the desk to see Dr. Woodrum with notes in hand from Dr. Kwon. By the time the notes were entered into the scheduling system, Dr. Woodrum was called into surgery consultation, otherwise we would have been in front of him in fifteen minutes. When he returned, he reviewed our scans, Dr. Kwon's notes, and conferred with his assessment. Cryoablation surgery (freezing) would be an appropriate and well tolerated treatment for this disease. After answering questions, we were scheduled for surgery the following Monday. This being Thursday, we also had pre-surgery appointments to be handled, which were made for Friday. Blood workups and an EEG all came back clean and the 5:45 am Monday surgery was confirmed.

All during this timeframe, there was an impending hurricane, Irma, heading toward Florida. With the advanced prediction capability getting better and better, along with the warning systems, we found ourselves connected to the news reports. "The hurricane is expected to make landfall and track over Tampa" (near our home) were words we did not want to hear. We were helpless in our ability to do anything in preparation for its arrival. Stuck in Rochester, Minnesota, talking to our friends and family, and praying for intervention was extremely stressful.

The storm was expected to strike on Saturday and my sister, who was weathering out the storm, managed to go to our house and secure it as much as possible. All we could do then was to wait for the report to see if we still had a home left when it passed. We both agreed that staring at the news did nothing for our well-being, so we decided to take a trip on Saturday to Winona, Minnesota as a distraction.

It was a beautiful late summer day with just a hint of a chill in the morning air. On the drive to Winona, we traversed over gentle rolling plains and farmlands as the sun brought its rays of warmth into the car. The road would wind gently back and forth, bringing an occasional farmhouse into view where the cattle would be calmly grazing on the grasses. Once closer to Winona, which sits on the shore of the Mississippi River, we began the descent into the river valley. It is humbling to see the evidence of the power of water as you make your way down to the valley level. There is only an elevation change of seven hundred feet, but that is enough to have created large cuts in the land where the centuries of rain water has made its way to the river. Once at the river level, the town of Winona with about twenty thousand residents appears as a peaceful place.

As we drove into the outskirts of the city, we passed through an industrial section that was adjacent to the inland waterways of the river. There were channels that allowed the barges to moor and load their cargo from the shoreline silos. This obviously was a grain port where the surrounding farmlands brought their bounty for shipment to the world. As we moved through the area, we noticed a sign alongside the road, "Maritime Art Museum." While we were not big on the maritime component, we always have been drawn to art. After a brief "You wanna go?" "Sure, you wanna go?" discussion, we turned around and headed back. Entering the parking lot, we found only a couple of cars there. We parked and strolled toward the building, enjoying the now warmer pre-fall day. There was a set of gardens surrounding the building and a path leading down toward the water. The flowers were perfect places for bees to be gathering their last-minute nectar before the snow begins to fly, so, avoiding the bees, we gingerly made our way to the front doors.

As we entered, we were greeted by two elderly women

159

who sat patiently behind the reception counter. "Welcome to our museum, it's $7.00 per person!" one said matter of factly. We decided it would serve as a great distraction to our Florida home dilemma, so I reached into my pocket and paid the lady who told us there were six galleries and to take our time and enjoy. The first gallery was full of very tastefully displayed photographs that represented all aspects of the Mississippi River. These encompassed all seasons and all locations of the Mississippi, including from its mouth in Louisiana to its origin in Minnesota. The photographs were not what we were expecting, although I am not exactly sure what I was expecting. Some were excellent expressions of colors of the flowers and sun, while others focused more on the textures of the frozen ice. All were stunningly beautiful in their own way.

Next, we moved into the "European Gallery." Pausing before passing through the "VAULT" doors, we began to wonder, "What kind of place is this?" Entering, we were faced with masterpieces from Monet (my personal favorite), Renoir, Van Gogh, Da Vinci and more , all excellently displayed. The gallery curator sat at the desk next to the entrance and welcomed us with the inclusion of "If you have any questions, feel free to ask."

Another visitor couple was casually and quietly moving from piece to piece. The room was silent, except for the occasional gasp when they moved to the next piece. The paintings were hung on the walls with little barrier to their access. You could walk up to a masterpiece and almost touch your nose to the print. At times, you would anticipate catching a whiff of the paint as it dried. We could marvel in the close-up intricacies of the artist's hand and trace the brushstrokes, following their creative technique.

The curator occasionally came by and added little bits of detail regarding the artist, the location, or the subject. We moved from piece to piece, repeating our predecessors in their gasps as a new marvelous revelation appeared before us. At one point, I was standing in front of two Van Goghs, one from early in his career and the other from late. The progression of his art and his mental state were remarkable. As I was admiring the latter, the curator came up to me and pointed across the room to a painting we had not seen yet and exclaimed, "You see that painting over there? The guy that painted it was crazy." I looked across the room, looked back at the Van Gogh and then to him.

Lifting my arms toward the Van Gogh, I said, "Do you see the irony of standing in front of an artist's work who was certified crazy and exclaiming that that guy was crazy?"

He smiled sheepishly and said, "That is kind of funny, isn't it?" and walked away snickering.

The gallery of the European Masters was by far the one that made the most impression on both of us. The other galleries, while equally spectacular, just seemed a step down from after experiencing the masterpieces in the European Master Gallery. I almost wish we would have walked it in the reverse order. The appreciation and anticipation would have grown incrementally, allowing us to fully take in the others before experiencing the greats. Again, do not get me wrong. There were original masterpieces I would be proud to claim in all the galleries, but it was hard to move from a place of excellence to a place of acceptable. This is why we find ourselves increasingly frustrated by the medical profession outside of the Mayo circle. When you know there is a standard that can be met, and it is not, then disappointment abounds.

Leaving the museum, having been fully blessed, we made our way to the riverfront where we found a quaint restaurant nestled next to the water. Their claim to fame was definitely their location. Thank goodness because their food was mediocre at best. The view, however, was great. We found a sense of peace, looking over the river and its activities while we caught glimpses of the hurricane weather reports on the tv monitors. As we were enjoying the view and gaining some nourishment, we struck up a conversation with a couple sitting next to us who were also observing the weather reports. When they asked us where we were from, we simply pointed at the TV and exclaimed "There." It was ironic because at that very moment the image on the TV was directly over our neighborhood. They simply shook their heads, gave us well wishes, and went about their meal. What could you really say?

Next, we made our way up to a lookout point high above the valley. Once there, the true scope of the Mississippi River Valley became apparent. Below was the town nestled gently against the river. In front of it were two lakes formed when the river channel long ago changed direction leaving these oblong bodies of water in its absence. On the other side of the river rose the banks of Wisconsin back up to the original elevation, matching the Minnesota side. From our vantage point, it was approximately two plus miles across. To the south you could follow the valley toward Lacrosse for what appeared to be fifteen miles, and to the north toward the cities it was another fifteen miles. After that the valley turned, revealing only the high banks. All in all, it was very impressive. It is life-giving water that has scoured the earth away, washing it eventually toward the Gulf of Mexico where it lays it to rest, building the deltas. Mother Nature again displays her majesty.

The drive back to Mayo seemed relaxing. Full of renewed energy from the day's wonders, we arrived back in town in time to secure an evening meal and immerse ourselves back into reality. We learned through various sources that our home and community had been spared the brute force of the hurricane. Irma decided to track further east than expected and, except for an occasional tree coming down, all was spared. After saying a prayer of thanks, we retired to bed for a good night's rest and to contemplate the upcoming procedure. I would like to say it was restful bliss, but that would be a lie. The surgery was straight forward and our confidence in the doctors was strong. But, anytime you go under anesthesia, there are assumed risks. Not being willing to dwell on the "what ifs?" I have trained myself to focus on the "why nots?" In doing so, I drifted off to slumber land, believing the procedure would be a total and complete success. After all, why not?

We spent Sunday getting caught up on some of our workload and a little bit of shopping. For me, it was the inclusion of comfortable clothes for both the time in the hospital and the expected eight hour drive the following day. The next morning, bright and early, we were off to the hospital for the surgery. Arriving at zero dark fifteen,

163

we checked into the appointment and immediately were whisked to the pre-op area. There, an IV was inserted, patient attire donned, forms filled out, and a patient video viewed. Next, off we went to the prep room where we chatted and prayed about the procedure while we waited for the staff to take me to the operating room (OR).

Around 7:30 am, they came and took me away down the halls, but not before Marilyn and I said our customary "I love you," which I take much more seriously now. Not that I have ever said these words to her idly, it is more that our love is growing more deeply than before. That seems odd to say, implying that it was not that before, but God has taught me that there is an unlimited supply of love and that there is always more to be acquired and given.

Inside the OR, the attending staff was buzzing around the room. "Please tell me your name and birth date." "What are you here for?" "Where are we doing the procedure?" All these questions were blurred in with the preparations surrounding me. Eventually my focus came to one person, the anesthesiologist, who was getting ready to begin the process. "Mr. Fuller, I am going to begin injecting the anesthetic into your IV. You will feel a little coolness in your arm...." This was immediately followed by "Welcome back! How are you feeling? Here, take a little drink."

The silence after that was broken only by the beeping of the heart monitors pulsing in the background. Little did I know that it was five plus hours later, and I was in a hospital room with Marilyn by my side. It takes a little while to come out of the fog, even more so with the pain medication I was being given. However, I was alert enough when the doctor came in and filled us in on the procedure. "Everything went well. We drilled three holes into your hip bone approximately four inches deep and froze the affected areas. We monitored the nerve activity during the procedure and the neurologist is confident there is no nerve degradation or damage. Everything went well." The rest of the day entailed me drifting in and out of sleep, requesting additional pain medications and talking to Marilyn and the staff. They brought a cot into the room, so Marilyn could stay with me during the night. In and out of sleep, it was comforting knowing she was within eyeshot. I do Love this woman!

The next day we were released around noon. We made our way to the pharmacy near the lobby, picked up my medications, and then went out the door to the car in the parking garage. I found a sitting position that felt tolerable and off we went. Our intention was to see how far I could bear to travel and then get a hotel to rest. Fortunately, with the pain medication's help, we were able to make the entire nine-hour trip. Arriving at our son's house, it was good to again get horizontal. The pain radiated from my back, where they made the incisions, to the hip bone and surrounding tissue.

The doctor had described the procedure well, letting us know that when they apply the freezing force, there will be a margin of error outside of the targeted bone. This area of muscle and nerve will experience the same damage as frostbite. Muscle and nerves will heal and, as a part of that process, there will be pain. This will diminish over time and all will return to normal, so be patient, use the prescribed medications, and enjoy life. The evening rest was welcome and, with the inclusion of the pain medication, I was able to sleep soundly. The next morning, I was able to get up and go into work for a few hours. Again, there is a sense of peace in that routine.

We stayed in Indiana through the month of September and decided we would return to Florida in October. This time we would drive to Florida instead of flying so we could pull a trailer back later with things for our new northern home. Another reason we were staying around in Indiana, was because a dear friend of ours had gone through prostate cancer treatment around the same time as I, and he was experiencing some health challenges. We wanted to be close to him and his family and offer whatever assistance we could.

We also had a new Indiana home to continue to get ready for our return. To us, the logic made sense and we settled back into our routine. My pain began to subside, and I dropped off the pain medications quickly. Not being one to wallow in misery, I would work during the day and then go to the house to paint and prep. Climbing up and down a ladder did present challenges, but I would be cautious and stop whenever the pain would intensify. We managed and at the end of September, off we went on our twelve-hundred mile trek.

Arriving in Florida, we went about determining what would go north and what would stay. Also, we decided that it was time to update the Florida home because we had not really made it ours when we bought it back in 2014. Our routine looked something like this, work on our computers for six to eight hours, sort through the house, shop for furniture we would take north, shop for design details for the southern home, meet with contractors and, most definitely, spend time with family and friends. All of this with the knowledge that we were returning to Indiana the first of November for my wife's family Christmas. Throw in there a scheduled blood test to check the status of my PSA to confirm the success of the mitigation surgery. It didn't seem like an uncomfortable schedule, but writing it down now makes me tired.

Mayo was adamant that we should maintain consistency in our testing. Although PSA tests are universal, there is a slight discrepancy in the results based on equipment calibration. With the possible recurrence of prostate cancer looming after the surgery, they wanted to maintain that level of control. They had arranged to send out a test kit for having the blood locally drawn and then returning it to their laboratory for evaluation. Everything was going well, and when the blood test kit arrived, we made the appointment to have it drawn.

At this same time, our friend was taking a turn for the worse. He had developed Leukemia from a weakened immune system from his radiation treatment of the bone. He was seeking medical attention for its treatment and had finally scheduled his first rounds of Chemo when he came down with pneumonia. This complicated the treatment plan and after admission to the hospital, they attempted to give him his first treatment. It did not go well, and the prognosis looked dreary.

At this same time, we checked the patient portal at Mayo the day after my blood test and found my PSA had climbed significantly. It was now at 56, its highest level ever. Red flags went off and we were immediately on the phone with the clinic. "Please have Dr. Kwon review the blood work and contact us at his earliest convenience." Advising us that he was in clinic all day, they assured us that he was scheduled to review the results tomorrow and contact us then.

The following day, we received a message through the portal to contact them immediately. Making the call, we were informed that they had written orders for me to have additional bloodwork done and a new C-11 PET scan. "How soon could we be back in Rochester?" This was a Wednesday and, since we were driving to Indiana, we confirmed that we could be there on Tuesday the following week. The appointments were set and now we were working on an accelerated timeline. Rent the trailer, cancel appointments, schedule a time to load, notify family and friends, and more became our focus.

On top of this, we found out that our Indiana friend was still not doing well, and they were transferring him to hospice. It is painful to be away from loved ones when you know they are suffering. Not that our presence would have changed the outcome, but more to be comforters to them and they to us. Still we had to stay focused.

Pushing through the obstacles, we were packed and ready to go by Friday evening. Leaving first thing in the morning pulling a trailer, we headed out with determination. We were now not only going for my medical needs; we were going to a funeral for our friend who had succumbed to the disease as well as to support his family. The trip north was uneventful, albeit slower than usual. The trailer held us back and used a lot of gas. We drove for fourteen hours and managed to make it to Bowling Green, Kentucky before we called it quits. Up and at it the next morning, we pulled into our northern home around 3:30 in the afternoon. Our cousin came over and helped us unload the trailer before we made our way to our son's home.

Marilyn made a call to our friend's wife to check in, and she immediately invited us to come over. Gladly, we went to spend some time with her and her family. Leaving with hugs and tears, we went to our welcoming bed for a much anticipated, albeit short rest. The viewing and funeral were to be the next day, Monday.

The next morning it was off to work, drop off the trailer, and head to the viewing. The funeral followed, and we said our goodbyes before departing for Mayo. We drove until 11 pm and checked into a hotel. Up the next morning, we finished the drive and arrived in Rochester around noon. Plenty of time to rest, get a little work done and make our way over to the clinic for blood draws and scans. Wednesday morning, we checked out of the hotel and made our way to the appointment.

Dr. Kwon was somewhat taken back. The C-11 PET scan had indicated there was widespread metastatic disease in various places on my bones. The treated areas continued to remain clear, but this presented a new dynamic to the treatment process. Clearly, there is a need to change strategies and his recommendation to move toward a more systemic treatment plan indicated we were moving into yet another action phase. We discussed the options and agreed that the next phase would take us down a path that included chemo and hormone therapy. The decision of where we would begin this treatment was entirely ours. During our time before this appointment, we had discussed our options in case this was a recommended path. Having learned that where you begin your chemo treatments becomes the place you stay for the duration, we had decided that Florida would be the appropriate place.

If I was going to be braving through chemo cycles where you feel good, then bad, then good, I preferred to be where it is warm, so if I felt well enough, I could enjoy the outdoors. Also, Marilyn's support system in Florida would be more available to her. Not that there is not the support in Indiana, it's about the availability. So, the decision was made, and we were now off on our drive back to Indiana, which went from snow, to slush, to dry conditions, eventually to rain, then to pouring rain.

During this ever-changing drive, Marilyn was on the phone with various doctors' offices in Florida, conferring the urgency and making appointments. In conjunction to this, she was checking and booking airline flights for me to Florida. (Marilyn would be staying behind in Indiana to help with the preparations for our family Christmas. My intent was to go to Florida, get the first treatment, and return immediately to Indiana. As much as we were going through this together, I felt this was something I could handle alone.) By the end of the nine-hour drive, we had flight reservations for Thursday and doctor appointments on Friday. Again, we got back to our bed at 10:30 that evening and I was flying out a mere thirteen hours later.

Arriving in Florida, I went to the doctor's office to verify the appointment and provide them with any missing documentation. I was able to overcome a couple of obstacles with the insurance during that visit and cleared the way for the next day's appointments. The following day,

I met with our now chosen hematologist. He had reviewed the scans and agreed with Dr. Kwon on the treatment plan. The issue was now timing. He indicated that we could get the Lupron (hormone deprivation drug) administered by Friday next week and then set the appointments for the Taxotere (Chemo) infusion the following week.

I politely and respectfully said, "No!" I was flying back out of Florida to Indiana on Thursday the following week for a family Christmas and needed all of this accomplished by Wednesday. We discussed the obstacles to this and agreed it could be done. We, the doctor, his staff, and I, divided up the responsibilities and set the appointments. Then we waited for Monday's new beginning.

Chapter 10

Let the Journey Continue

I arrived at the clinic for the afternoon blood draw and orientation meeting with mixed emotions. First was the feeling of getting this chapter started and heading toward a cure, and second was the feeling of apprehension.

Chemo is a series of drugs and their supporting elements, which are designed to kill you. Now granted, properly administered they will kill the bad cancer cells more quickly, which allows them to be beneficial. Finding the correct dose to maintain that balance between life and death has been a testament to the medical staff and their patients who have gone before. Most importantly, it was the patients who were fully invested in the process. In some cases, these individuals made quality-of-life versus length-of-life choices. Chemo will weaken you and can make your remaining time miserable. On the other hand, the prognosis without chemo would be a more aggressive disease and shortened life. Risk the side effects or wait to die. That decision would have been a difficult one and a test of their faith.

As mentioned earlier, years ago, back in 1972, my brother Mike passed away from leukemia. He was serving in the Navy when the diagnosis was made shortly after he had just married the love of his life. The disease had progressed undetected. At the time it was discovered, he was in advanced stages and was only given days to live. His decision to receive cutting edge, unproven treatment back then was a mostly unselfish act. Now, the wanting to live is strong, but so is the desire to make lives better for others.

These new "chemo" drugs were just in their infancy and the dosages were yet unknown. Too little would have insignificant effects and contribute to the misery. Too much would certainly kill you. Somewhere in the balance, it was suspected, there was a chance at life. Unfortunately, these technologies did not come with pre-written instruction manuals, and the only way to determine their success was to try.

As he progressed through the various stages of the treatments, there were successes and there were failures. The inevitable roller coaster he and his new bride, along with his loving family, went on was an emotional journey. One day there would be progress, the next regression. Next came feelings of well-being which were followed by desires to die. In the end, he lost the battle and succumbed to death, but not before contributing to the scientific community, holding his newborn daughter, and building them a home to keep them warm. My love and appreciation along with the gratitude for him and the other pioneers grows stronger as I understand their sacrifices.

Back to my story, the nurse welcomed me and escorted me to the blood draw room. There, blood was drawn, analyzed, and the report handed back to me. Next, we shuffled to the "Infusion Room" where the orientation would take place. A brief tour of the facility and introductions to some of the staff was followed by, "Have a seat and we will let you know what your next few months will most likely look like." The nurse was a very meticulous individual who left no stone unturned. Starting at the beginning, we covered the progression of drugs, their administration, and the potential side effects. Each drug has side effects. The drugs used to counteract the side effects have side effects and on and on.... The conversation had to come to a close somewhere and through experience she simply stated, "We will address that, if needed," and then moved to the next topic.

My treatment was scheduled for the following day, so she covered what that would be like. Treatment time would be around two hours with little to do but read or pass the time in your own way. As I glanced around, there were others receiving their scheduled doses. Some were lying back in the heated chair with a blanket, resting quietly. Others were working on a crossword or reading a book. Some were just staring into space with whatever thoughts milling around in their heads.

I left that appointment with a plethora of documentation on the drugs to be administered during the session. There were seven drugs used to support the treatments, along with controlling the potential side effects. Next was a trip to the local pharmacy to stock up on supplies and to continue on the quest of insurance clarification. As fate would have it, our insurance policies had renewed during this time and the transfer of data, or mostly lack thereof, created a new set of challenges. The databases had not been updated and all claims were being rejected due to deductibles and out-of-pocket amounts not being satisfied. There is a big difference between knowing what problem exists and identifying a solution versus being able to actually correct the problem. My role would simply be keeping it in front of the individuals with authority and their systems to facilitate the needed changes. Again, this area of patience and waiting prevails.

On the day of the treatment, my sister escorted me to the clinic. She was allowed to come back to the infusion room and provided a source of comfort and conversation. Everyone receives chemo differently, so there were some unknowns going into this.

Settling into the chair, turning on the heat, and waiting for the nurse to begin the process, I quietly observed the others sharing this journey with me. As mentioned before, I found it interesting how each person addressed the treatments. It left me wondering what was their state of mind? Some seemed indifferent to the process. They sat quietly absorbed in the activity of their choice, patiently waiting for the infusion to be over, so they can go about the process of dealing with the side effects. Others were nervously knitting, crocheting, or reading, simply passing the time. Were they thinking that this was a path to healing or a process of dying? I believe that there was a little of both present in the room.

The nurse arrived at my station with the cart full of goodies. She proceeded to review the events which will unfold while carefully cleaning and prepping the infusion site. For me, it was on the inside of my arm. After inspecting the site, she carefully guided the needle for the IV into my arm, taking care to ensure it was properly placed in a vein and had sufficient flow for the chemo drug. After flushing the IV, she hung a bag of saline and began a slow drip to begin hydration. During the hydration phase, she came back to inject a drug into the IV. First was a drug which helps with the effects of nausea. After a dwell time, she returned to administer another drug which lessens the pain of the infusion. Only after these had been processed did she return to hang the "chemo" drug on the tree of hopefully life.

Slowly, the drug dripped out of the bag into my IV. As most people will testify, I have unique thoughts about most things. As I watched the drips fall into the liquid below, I was struck at the simplicity of the system. Poke a hole in your body, pour in some liquid, and wait to see what happens. The technology of the drug was also moving though my inquisitive brain. Who would have thought to create a chemical that would break the DNA of your cells to prevent them from replicating? But, only to the degree that they would allow the natural forces of our wonderfully made bodies the time to repair that DNA and allow slow dividing cells a chance to live.

Then came the thought of, what is next? Little side effects would show up on the first day, but what about tomorrow? A fleeting thought also made its way through my brain, "I wonder if I will lose my hair?" But, mostly, it was simply a time to wait until the infusion was over. Then my sister and I unceremoniously left the clinic and returned home. There, I quietly went about the remainder of a usual day.

The evening was uneventful. I felt a slight bit of nausea, but nothing concerning. My rest was normal, and even the night's sleep was uneventful. In the morning, I arose wondering what would be different and began my day. This day, like every day following chemo, I would need to return to the clinic for an injection of a drug named Neulasta. This drug is designed to counteract one of the side effects of the chemo which causes your bones to slow, or stop, producing white and red blood cells. The absence of these will greatly compromise your ability to fight the effects of the chemo. This drug revs up the bone marrow, causing it to go into overdrive.

The injection was simple: a tiny needle, a poke, and a little bandage. The side effects of this on the following day were highly under rated. I do not know how else to describe it but to say your bones hurt, a lot, from the inside out. There was no place on me you could touch. Everything hurt. This lasted for a couple of days and then everything began to settle down.

After the Neulasta injection, the next thing on the agenda was to prepare to return to Indiana for our family Christmas. Full of drugs that were now working to kill me slowly enough to allow the healthy cells to survive, I boarded the plane and flew back to Indiana, back to Marilyn. I know this sounds a little crazy. Everyone reacts differently, and to distance myself from the caregivers after the first infusion was maybe not the smartest decision. My reasoning was that if I were to allow cancer to run my life, I would become a slave to it, giving it power over my life. I needed to maintain control for as long as I could. Going about my life by celebrating Christmas with our loved ones could only bring power and comfort. How could I possibly not do this? I am so thankful that I have these loving, supporting souls in my life. For now, I will fully enjoy today and see what tomorrow brings, tomorrow. After the Christmas celebration, we boarded a plane together and flew back to Florida.

The next couple of weeks were mostly uneventful. Slight nausea, weakness, and fatigue were present but manageable. On the thirteenth day things changed. Not in the above side effects but in the shower. That morning, I stepped into the shower and began the routine. First was to wash my hair and rinse the shampoo. This time there was something different. After rinsing my hair, I realized that the shampoo was still in my hair and felt it running down my face. Sticking my head back under the shower, I rinsed again with the same results. After the third time, I let the water clear only to look down and see my hair running toward the drain. My first instinct was to laugh followed by a call to Marilyn to come look. Being the sensitive person she most certainly is, she pulled back the curtain, looked down and began laughing with me.

What Marilyn did next took me a little off guard. "Wait, I'll be right back," she said as she left the bathroom. Returning with phone in hand she proceeded to point the camera into the shower.

"Careful, I'm naked" was all I could manage to say as she began to take pictures of the hair on the floor. Thank goodness for her discretion or this could be a different kind of story. Reaching up to my head, I could grab handfuls and simply pull hair out. Knowing how this was going to end up, after I got out of the shower and dressed, I called my hair gal and had her take all of it off. Now, whatever may be left would only be tiny pieces instead of the long strands. Besides, it was somewhat liberating not having to wonder if it would all go.

Now completely bald, I continued on the journey. Twenty-one days later, I headed to the clinic for my next infusion. This process repeated without fail for a total of six sessions. Midway through the treatment sessions, there was a hurricane which devastated Puerto Rico. Not living in Puerto Rico, you would not think this would be a problem. Come to find out, the vast majority of the saline solution used in the United States is produced in Puerto Rico. Now facing shortages, the treatment infusions had to be adjusted. The chemo dosage did not change, only the amount of liquid used to deliver it and the length of time to run it into my body. This would not be disruptive to the treatment but would potentially affect the side effects, and it did. The sense of nausea intensified. The pain ratcheted up, and, more importantly for me, the ability to rest and sleep dropped significantly. Eventually, I found myself sleeping in the comfort of a recliner at night. It seemed to be the only place I could find some relief.

During this time, Marilyn's wings began to shine. She absolutely was an angel to me. I do not know how I deserved to find her in my life but am truly grateful for her love, presence, and companionship. Through the sleepless nights, I would hear her periodically checking in on me, making sure I was fine, seeing if I needed anything, and, more importantly, voicing concern. Sometimes it was a gentle touch to let me know she was there, other times it was simply being aware that she was in the room with me. In all cases, the feeling of Love was conveyed to someone who was not aware that it was needed at the time.

Also, during these times, I would wake up in the middle of the night immersed in thoughts. Most were simply idle and frivolous; others were thoughtful and deep. One night I slowly entered into consciousness with an awareness of a conversation I was having. It was not as though I woke up and started a conversation. It was simply that I found myself in the middle of an ongoing one. This conversation was with God. Lots of things were being discussed or conveyed, but the most important was the understanding that God had created me.

My understanding was, "David, I created Man in the perfect image of Myself—perfect and flawless in every way. As creators yourselves, Man, My perfect creation, took it upon himself to create of himself something beyond My design and then identified fully with it with all its flaws and imperfections. Man left the perfect identity I gave him and turned his back on Me. Once you return to the you I created, you will again be perfect. Trust in this."

With that understanding, I was at complete peace. I knew, from the vision I was given before, coupled with the understanding that I have an unwavering relationship with God, that all will be well.

Chemo has an interesting way of interacting with our bodies. I spoke with others who were going though similar treatments, and they described some of their side effects. One gentleman said that his body ached shortly after the infusion. He would then get extremely cold and even

181

though the temperature in the house was 80-plus degrees, he still needed to sit with a cover over him no matter what. Another guy stated that he became very nauseous. Most times when he attempted to eat, it would only take a few bites and then he would throw up. Knowing that he needed to keep up his strength, he would return to the table and try it again. Most times the process would repeat. Eventually, he was able to keep enough down to sustain life. A third gentleman simply stated that he slept. After taking in the infusion, he would wait a day or two and then all facets of energy drained from his body, leaving him recused to the recliner. After several days, he would begin to gain some energy back and find some semblance of a normal life.

I, on the other hand, tolerated the chemo very well. Energy was mostly good, an occasional nap when needed, well mostly daily, and my appetite and tolerance was normal. There was one very unusual side effect . I had this lingering taste of butter in my mouth. Everything I ate had an aftertaste of butter. Ice cream, steak, tacos, cereal, nothing was spared. I told my wife, "The good news is I don't have to butter the toast in the morning." We and our friends both had a fun time with that and still do to this day.

Four years after the first elevated PSA test, chemo was over. I had managed to survive the treatments and their effects without serious complications. Now began the after-chemo regiment. The doctors prescribed Lupron injections quarterly and a daily oral chemo drug named Zytiga, which required a dose of Prednisone. This was followed up by a quarterly injection of Xgeva. Each of these had specific purposes, and combined, the doctors felt they would work to kill any remaining cancer cells which may have dodged the chemo.

My physical state at this time was weakened. The further into the treatments, the less energy the chemo drugs left me. Even though I attempted to get some exercise, I could tell that my body was weakened. Marilyn would encourage me to get out and do something during the chemo treatments. This involved walks in the neighborhood, going out with friends, and the occasional journey to our community "Happy Hour." There, I could connect with friends, enjoy some music, and indulge in an occasional slow dance with the Love of my life. The result of these activities was at times weariness or total exhaustion. Even so, it kept me active and connected to a life I could only, at times, dream of.

Now, with the chemo over, I felt I had a chance to return to a routine which involved "getting healthy again." It is funny thinking of it in this way because the entire process was for this purpose. But somehow, ending chemo treatments felt like a line in the sand. We did not know what the results of the chemo would be. There is a chance that the treatments simply slowed the progress of the cancer. There was a chance it did nothing.

We, I, believed that it was successful in its intent and killed "all" of the cancer completely. This is where faith comes in, and the thought of anything short of a cure seemed disappointing. So, the idea that these new drugs were even needed brought in that moment of doubt that we all experience at times. I have always been someone who trusts in God and recognizes that the medical breakthroughs are simply God's wisdom expressed in human form. Therefore, my expectations from the treatments would be positive but precautionary until the final statement of remission or cure could be claimed. Doubt would simply be a fleeting thought which has no power in my life.

The after-chemo medications, Lupron, Zytiga, and Xgeva, all have a component of fatigue as a side effect. Knowing that my true self would remain hidden for a while, we began the new series of treatments. Fatigue was definitely present but I knew that Marilyn truly wanted to get back to the Florida life we had begun. Not wanting to disappoint her, I sometimes just did things anyway. Despite the overwhelming desire to rest, we just enjoyed life. The walks became more frequent and longer in length, the socializing increased, and we planned more trips. It is not that the tiredness and fatigue got less, it was more that we were not going to let it rule our lives.

There were times that I simply said no. A day at home, resting or napping while watching a favorite show felt wonderful. Tomorrow would bring another day, and we would begin to reinsert ourselves into life. As time went on, my strength began to return. The side effects of the drugs were not so confining anymore. I do not know if my body was adjusting or if my attitude was. Maybe both at times. Either way, the idea of living with challenges simply did not matter. The fact was we were living again.

Four months after the end of chemo, we returned to Mayo Clinic. The routine was already established. Blood work to determine blood health and PSA numbers. An MRI to look for recurring metastasis and a C-11 scan to identify traces of cancer which may be left over from the chemo treatment. The blood work looked normal albeit a little weakened. The PSA was undetectable mostly because of the Lupron. If there had been a detectable PSA then we would have been confident that a significant amount of disease remained, but nothing. The MRI was clear with no new abnormalities found. They expected to see past abnormalities, however the evidence of nothing new was promising.

Finally, the results of the C-11. "No evidence of metastatic disease" was the news we were looking for and expected and gratefully received. Considering the place where we came from prior to chemo, Dr. Kwon simply stated, "You are doing great." Those words, spoken from one of the best prostate cancer doctors in the world, were working their way into our heads. Could it be? Were we? Was I finally on the final leg of this journey? Needless to say, we were elated by the news. Dr. Kwon followed up with the statement, "We just need to stay the course and follow up in three months." The drugs would continue, and we would keep a watchful eye on any signs of any progression of the cancer.

The reality of cancer is that you never fully escape its grip on your life. As the successive reports continued to come in with "great" news, I am still constantly aware that there could be a relapse sometime in my future. Dr. Kwon stated it in this way, "You will always have cancer cells in your body. The question is whether they are alive or dead. Only through the active diligence of maintenance drugs and routine scans will that answer be known." So, for now, I will maintain the regiment of drugs prescribed. In time, as the tests continue to return "great" reports, we will look at removing them from my life. Today and in my future, I will live every day with the gratitude and understanding that I have come to a place where many cancer patients only hope to be. I'm thankful for all that has been given to me, both the good and the bad, for it was through each that God revealed Himself in amazing ways while simply wanting me to "Go for a walk with Him."

Let the Journey continue!